Theory and Method in a
Study of Argentine Fertility

Theory and Method in a Study of Argentine Fertility

AARON V. CICOUREL

A WILEY-INTERSCIENCE PUBLICATION

JOHN WILEY & SONS, New York • London • Sydney • Toronto

Library of Congress Cataloging in Publication Data:

Cicourel, Aaron Victor, 1928-
    Theory and Method in a study of Argentine fertility.
    "A Wiley-Interscience publication."
    Bibliography: p.

    1. Fertility. 2. Argentine Republic—Population.
3. Social surveys. I. Title.

HB903.F4C44   301.32'1'0982   73-14985
ISBN 0-471-15793-7

Printed in the United States of America

10 9 8 7 6 5 4 3 2 1

My research in Argentina was motivated by several interests. I wanted to pursue methodological and theoretical issues described in previous writings in a comparative context. I felt that these methodological and theoretical issues should be pursued in a different area—for example, fertility—to show the breadth of earlier ideas applied to education and deviance. I wanted to demonstrate how notions of everyday social interaction are presupposed in the study of such macro issues as differences in fertility rates. Finally, I wanted to initiate a long-standing (but still unrealized) interest in the study of Latin American social structure. I had no desire to become an "area" specialist, but I did want to immerse myself in a setting that would provide a useful comparative basis for pursuing methodological and theoretical issues explored heretofore only in an American context.

This book does not follow the usual sociological approaches to the study of fertility or Latin America. I try to do more than replicate important research on fertility in Jamaica (Blake 1961) and Puerto Rico (Stycos 1955) using modified survey methods. I try to address these issues by contrasting traditional theoretical and methodological approaches with the program described in my earlier work, *Method and Measurement in Sociology.* Hence I create traditional tables primarily to allow the reader to compare their interpretation with a textual analysis of the original interview materials. The tables, therefore, are relegated to a rather minor position in the study.

I begin with some general problems in demography and the substantive study of fertility that cross-cut the social organization of different societies. I discuss attempts to narrow the gap betwen these macro studies and the concern with social psychological aspects of fertility. A recent book by Beshers (1967) provides a social psychological perspective that enables me to outline my own contrasting views. Background information on Argentina is then supplied to enable the reader to locate the study ethnographically and historically. The remaining chapters describe the sample used for the study, presenting some findings, as well as a detailed discussion of how a textual analysis of the interview materials forces us to reexamine traditional research strategies and theoretical assumptions usually associated with surveys. An idea of the field conditions encountered is conveyed by a detailed picture of a few families. I have tried to stress the importance of understanding the social context within which the interviews were conducted and the larger problems in human information processing that these interviews create. These larger problems take us beyond the study of fertility and deal with important issues in all field research. The final chapter contains a brief outline of some new directions that are proposed for field research.

This is the first foreign study I have attempted. Fortunately, however, I had several friends, relatives, and acquaintances in Buenos Aires; this meant that I could obtain a native's view about my initial tourist-oriented observations and feel assured that the information I recorded would be checked for accuracy. Having these key informants in the local area, I could compare my more naïve initial impressions against those of natives, thereby avoiding mistakes a novice to foreign field work can make. But the contrasts also served to warn me how informants can filter out impressions that underline differences between groups within the country, and differences between Argentina and the United States.

My contacts enabled me to adjust more easily (but never completely) to changing views of my perceptions of a respondent's sincerity, as well as the interpretation of variations in local punctuality, "friendly" gestures, and the like. The verbal and nonverbal cues one is accustomed to in his native land and community are not the same in a foreign country, and they cannot be assumed to be the same if we are to recognize and describe comparative research problems.

Some of my difficulties began when I sought to recruit assistants. It took several weeks to discover that obtaining good interviewers meant crossing political and friendship lines and that it was important to guide training sessions carefully to prevent the opposing parties from using the time for their own arguments or disputes. On rare occasions, I felt pressured to take on and keep poor assistants (while assigning them less and less work) to maintain a viable research team.

Problems of comparative research became painfully obvious when I began, with the help of my friend Miguel Murmis, to translate the questionnaire. What I thought to be simple problems (how to say "flirting" without offending women respondents, yet maintaining colloquial usage when discussing with men their premarital contacts) turned out to be complicated. I was advised by assistants that it would be almost impossible to ask certain questions about sexual activities and the use of contraceptives, but I decided to push ahead nonetheless with a few pretests, and finally I convinced the group that the questions could be asked. My assistants felt that the questions were too personal for an Argentine sample and that a survey was not the best way to elicit information about sexual activities and the use of contraceptives.

My project was modestly financed and could not have been done if the Social Science Research Council (Joint Committee on Latin American Studies) had not given me its support. I received additional support from the University of California through half sabbatical pay and from the Institute of International Studies at Berkeley. The Institute of Sociology at the University of Buenos Aires provided funds for some secretarial help and helped pay part of my salary. The Population Council provided a small grant which enabled me to hire Ricardo Muratorio Posse at the International Population and Urban Research project at Berkeley. Mr. Muratorio did virtually all the coding operations, provided excellent suggestions about the quality of the materials, and constructed approximately two-thirds of the tables.

I am grateful to Judith Blake Davis for advice and the generous use of the questionnaire from her Jamaica study. I also received helpful advice from Kingsley Davis, Gino Germani, and William Petersen. In Buenos Aires, Miguel Murmis and Darío Canton were generous with their time and helpful advice. Nancy Lopez de Nisnovich proved to be a dedicated and outstanding administrative assistant, research assistant, and interviewer. She worked hard and was responsible for organizing the data. A number of persons helped me with the interviews and research assistance. I am grateful to Mable Arruñada, Elizabeth Balán, Anna Maria Caellas, Miriam Chorne, Santos Colabella, Estella Elbert, Marta Fernandez, Leticia Gurman, Adolfina Janson, Cristina Mendelarzu, Maria Luisa Salvarezza, Marta Slemanson, Juan Carlos Torre, Ponciano Torales, and Valentin. Margarita Sandoval proved to be an excellent typist when the questionnaire responses were placed on 5 × 8 cards. Mrs. Charlotte Williams typed most of the initial draft of the first five chapters of the manuscript from a messy handwritten copy. Pat Apodaca typed the remaining chapters of the first draft quickly and accurately. The last two drafts were typed with enthusiasm by Sue Miller, Beverly Strong, Jessica Diaz, and Becky Miller. I am grateful to Eric Valentine for insisting that I complete a careful reediting of the "final" draft of the manuscript, and to Martha Ramos for her very helpful editorial suggestions.

I also acknowledge the valuable assistance of the copy editor Brenda Griffing. I am responsible for the defects of the final version of the book.

Three interviewers were especially busy doing the majority of the interviews. The three—Estella Elbert, Leticia Gurman, and Maria Luisa Salvarezza—were very generous with their time and were exceptionally dedicated to my concern with field research problems. Santos Colabella did some intensive interviewing in a difficult suburban area where many had refused to participate in the study. In his attempt to discover the background of the resistance, he found a local "witch" and wrote me a very helpful report on the methodological problems he encountered.

I obtained a number of important interviews at the Children's Municipal Hospital because of the generosity of Dr. Florencio Escardó. Dr. Escardó made ward 17 availaible to me for intensive interviews with mothers coming from the shantytowns of Buenos Aires.

I found the study difficult, but it surely would have been impossible had it not been for those just mentioned and many, many others who remain anonymous to protect their identity. Finally, I want to acknowledge the careful research assistance of my wife Merryl, and her devoted patience and understanding throughout a difficult year.

AARON V. CICOUREL

University of California, San Diego
La Jolla, California
July 1973

Contents

CHAPTER 1   THEORETICAL AND METHODOLOGICAL ISSUES IN STUDIES OF POPULATION AND FERTILITY   1

CHAPTER 2   TWO VIEWS OF DECISION-MAKING AND SOME CONSEQUENCES FOR FIELD STUDIES OF FERTILITY   15

CHAPTER 3   NOTES ON THE ARGENTINE HISTORICAL CONTEXT AND SOME ETHNOGRAPHIC IMPRESSIONS OF BUENOS AIRES   27

CHAPTER 4   SOME GENERAL CHARACTERISTICS OF THE STUDY   62

CHAPTER 5   METHODOLOGICAL ISSUES IN FIELD STUDIES   73

CHAPTER 6   THE METHODOLOGICAL CONTEXT OF SUBSTANTIVE ISSUES IN FERTILITY   90

CHAPTER 7   CONTRASTING PERSPECTIVES IN THE ANALYSIS OF MATERIALS   113

CHAPTER 8   TEXTUAL ANALYSIS OF INTERVIEW MATERIALS   141

CHAPTER 9   SOCIOLINGUISTIC FEATURES OF FERTILITY INTERVIEWS   162

CHAPTER 10   AN ALTERNATE APPROACH TO FIELD RESEARCH   195

REFERENCES   205

AUTHOR INDEX   209

SUBJECT INDEX   211

ix

THEORY AND METHOD IN A
STUDY OF ARGENTINE FERTILITY

CHAPTER 1

THEORETICAL AND METHODOLOGICAL ISSUES
IN STUDIES OF POPULATION AND FERTILITY

The study of fertility is often linked to the population problem—the relation between numbers of people and their social and economic resources. This study is restricted to the procreative activities of women, primarily those who are or were married. I am less interested in the population problem than in what demographers and population analysts have to say about the causes of differences in fertility, and how such causes are attributed to social and economic conditions.

Demographers and population analysts often begin their discussions of fertility behavior by referring to what are believed to be facts, noting, for example, that underdeveloped areas usually have a much higher fertility rate than urbanized–industrial societies. They pay particular attention to establishing the point at which birth rates started to rise or fall and how rapidly the rise or fall occurred. The variables affecting the possibility of intercourse during the reproductive period, leading to the possibility of sexual behavior and pregnancy or the use of contraceptive techniques, are usually discussed as obvious influences on fertility rates. Factors mentioned are age of entrance into a marital or informal sexual union and the point at which the union was broken by divorce, desertion, separation, or death.

In the preceding paragraphs I used the terms "facts" and "variables" without placing quotation marks around them. Throughout this book, however, I often use such terms with quotation marks because it is seldom clear in studying human fertility how investigators incorporate their own and their respondents' decisions and inferences made during day-to-day activities, into the aggregated "facts" and designated "vari-

1

ables" usually cited as causally relevant. The present study seeks to narrow the methodological and substantive gap between the everyday activities of reproduction, and the demographic and population studies describing abstract relationships that cross-cut the social organization of different societies. The Indianapolis studies (Whelpton and Kiser 1958) helped narrow the gap by linking attitudes obtained from social surveys to abstract structural characteristics such as the age, sex, and occupational distributions of societies, and social mobility patterns, kinship, and gross measures of economic growth. But surveys designed to elicit information about process through attitudes, or about structure by asking factual questions, do not recognize adequately the importance of the interview setting. The interview settings often reify past experiences while simultaneously creating forms of social interaction that can exert independent influence on the manner of asking or paraphrasing questions and on the truncation or transformation of answers during the interview.

Recent studies of fertility have dealt with the micro level of analysis more carefully; the reliance on attitudinal surveys tends to prevail, however, despite important attempts to provide careful interviewing procedures and a textual analysis of responses (Stycos 1955; Stycos and Back 1964; Blake 1961; Rainwater 1960, 1965).

I became interested in fertility and family organization because I wanted to demonstrate the importance of linguistic and cognitive factors in the study of everyday social interaction. This chapter is restricted to a few traditional notions about fertility in industrial societies; it closes with a brief outline of the orientation I propose as an alternative to traditional approaches.

Recent Sociological Thought on Fertility. Discussions of fertility by Davis (1959), Petersen (1961), and Wrong (1967) have stated the issues well. In this section I want to summarize some of the relevant literature, subsequently focusing on an important paper by Davis (1963) to set the stage for my own observations on fertility and family organization.

There has been a great deal of speculation about the reasons for the decline in fertility rates in the Western nations during World War I and until the middle 1930s, and their increase in the late 1930s or early 1940s and into the 1960s. Out of this curiosity have come a number of studies of psychological motivations and social determinants affecting reproductive behavior. The decline and rise of fertility has been linked to trends in urbanization, changes in the mobility of social classes, and changes in family structure and function, attitudes, and motives.

Because of variations in reproduction within a given family over the woman's childbearing years, it became necessary to examine a number of factors—for example, the age at which persons marry, the decision to postpone having children, and how couples might change their attitudes and motives before and after having had one or more children. Researchers also examined differential fertility across different types of grouping (e.g., by designations of religion, rural or urban residence, race, occupation, income, or education, or by composite measures leading to statements about social class differences). Scholars have considered the reproductive intentions of couples before and after the birth of each child. The study of couples' intentions has led to the view that each birth must be examined in its particular social setting and the local circumstances deemed to be associated with reproduction (Westoff, Potter, Sagi, and Mishler 1961; Westoff, Potter, and Sagi 1963).

Many scholars have stressed the importance of demographic factors in assessing differential fertility rates, in contrast to the decisions leading to marriage and one or more children. The factors often cited include separating changes in the sex ratio (i.e., an increase in the number of women), the age at marriage and the number of women marrying, an apparent growth in the number of married women bearing a first child, and the number of births per mother (Petersen 1961: 239). Yet many researchers would agree with Wrong's statement that the decline in the fertility rates of Western countries is due to voluntary causes and is ". . . the result of deliberate restrictions on procreation consciously practiced by modern populations" (1967: 53–54). Hence the decline of fertility in Western populations is not simply a function of chemical and mechanical methods of contraception, and abolishing such methods would not lead to a rapid increase in the birth rate (Wyon 1963: 88; Wrong 1967: 57). The social scientist is interested in differential fertility because of the relation between types of families and the social structures within which they are created. This interrelationship has been described as the ". . . social usages governing (a) the conditions of marriage and (b) family behavior patterns that can affect the relative frequency of conception and childbearing" (Petersen 1961: 563).

Recent work on fertility has focused on nonindustrialized countries because of their declining mortality and high reproduction rates. Many of these studies have been concerned with the impact of fertility on economic development and with the possibility of changing reproductive patterns.

In discussing fertility studies in nonindustrialized areas, Davis (1959: 322–323) underscores a number of problems. For example, how do we arrive at the social conditions behind fertility? How do we deal with the ambiguity of the verbal statements elicited, and what do they mean in terms of our understanding of past and future behavior and reproductive decision-making in the context of different birth order? Additional factors cited by Davis include the discrepancy between normative and actual behavior, inappropriate categories for elicting information because of culture-bound problems, and the tendency to restrict such studies to limited contacts with the respondents. We could add to the foregoing list, but the difficulties noted will indicate some of the issues involved in fertility studies.

Wrong (1967: 62) has questioned whether we can compare a decline in mortality and fertility in the West to possibly similar declines in non-Western or Western countries with low industrialization, despite the case of Japan. Wrong's observation serves to reemphasize the importance of a culture area wherein a special "institutional arrangement" exists that is conducive to high fertility.

Many of the issues in the study of differential fertility can be clarified if we now examine more general topics in modern demograhic history.

Kingsley Davis is a sociologist who has spent much of his career emphasizing both micro- and macro-level aspects of social structures. I do not agree with the specific approaches he has used, nor with the way he has kept the micro and macro levels of analysis separate. However, Davis has done work which in several ways forms an exception to criticisms of fertility studies I describe in the next section.

In the paper "The Theory of Change and Response in Modern Demographic History" (1963), Davis provides a sophisticated sociological statement for explaining the data assembled by demographers. He confronts the analysis of macro data (aggregated statistical information) and offers a theoretical explanation of how social and behavioral activities could have produced the structural effects identified. He proposes what appear to be invariant stimulus conditions and response consequences to account for modern demographic history. Some of the problems associated with the process of demagraphic change and response are described in the following passage, (in which Davis is critical of the tendency of demographers to treat attitudinal or interactional factors as tacit rather than as central features of demographic outcomes (1963: 345):

One method of escape [from the "frightening complexity" of the process of demographic change and response] is to eschew any comprehensive theory, simply describing computations or working on a single hypothesis at a time. Another is to adopt some convenient over-simplification, such as the assumption that population is simply a matter of two capacities—a "reproductive urge" on the one side and "means of subsistence" on the other—or, at an opposite extreme, that demographic behavior is a function of a "traditional culture" or "value system."

A common practice of demographers is to use such terms as "society," "fertility," "abortion," "Japanese tolerance," and "West European beliefs," to reify or to anthropomorphize abstract collectivities or phenomena. Such truncated descriptive terms simplify and distort the complexities of everyday behavior. Calling the use of contraceptives or abortion a "response" to social and economic conditions leaves unexamined the paths by which the members of a group have come to perceive such conditions as "negative" in their everyday communication. Another practice is to avoid the study of the daily communicational activities of a group, yet to assume that such activities index or reflect demographic outcomes.

Davis notes that it is too simple to say that fertility eventually falls in response to a drop in mortality. (I am ignoring recent claims that fertility rates may have started to decline before a decline in mortality, for Davis's remarks are more general than these substantive claims.) The complexity of the claim is avoided when demographers ignore the kinds of information presupposed about how a decline would be noted by different members of a group and how respondents' social distribution of knowledge would be a central ingredient in making claims about the "perception" of a decline. The demographer fails to explain how the sustained natural increase resulting from a decline in mortality now would be seen as a "negative" sign or "stimulus," leading to collective responses that then lowered fertility.

The unexamined systems of communication and social settings embedded in different cultural arrangements which presumably lead to responses such as postponed marriage, the use of contraceptives, sterilization, abortion, and migration—are inferred in an interactional and cultural vacuum. Even when normative practices or accounts about cultural areas are used, or when the researcher simply makes use of his nativeness in asserting claims about demographic patterns in his own country, the sources of the information are not questioned, nor are they seen as ad hoc descriptions serving to sidestep the difficult issues rooted in the study of social interaction.

Davis's statement that "every country in northwest Europe reacted" to the excess of births over deaths makes reference to activities such as postponing marriage, emigrating overseas, obtaining abortions, practicing celibacy, and (to some extent) using contraceptives. The assumption made is that a "message" (that a decline in mortality was leading to sustained natural increase) was evident or perceived in different countries among various groups and individuals. The perception of the stimulus (excess births over deaths or sustained natural increase) was apparently "clear," but the "response" varied.

Davis's claim that a simplistic notion of poverty is inadequate to explain the "response" of lower fertility, despite a decline in mortality, is persuasive. He notes (Davis 1963: 351) that northwest Europeans and the Japanese were not "pushed" by growing poverty:

> The answer to the central question about modern demographic history cannot be posed, then, in the framework of ordinary population theory, which assumes the sole "population factor" to be some relation between the population–resources ratio and the collective level of living. It is doubtful that any question about demographic behavior can be satisfactorily posed in such terms, because human beings are not motivated by the population–resources ratio even when they know about it (which is seldom).

The appeal of this analysis lies in the author's continual references to realistic possibilities in the everyday life of the family and his suggestion that these contingencies could have produced the gross outcomes that demographers tend to oversimplify by avoiding explicit theorizing at the level of everyday family life. Let me outline some of the points made by Davis.

People in northwest Europe during the late nineteenth and early twentieth centuries, as well as the Japanese after World War II, somehow became aware that their customary demographic behavior was handicapping their efforts to take advantage of a changing economy. The link between a "changing" economy that offered new opportunities and a desire on the part of members to benefit from the changes is presumed by demographers to result in modifications in demographic behavior; such substantive claims are difficult to study historically at the level of day-to-day living, however, and they remain difficult to study in contemporary research. Theories about everyday life and the general structure of social interaction are presupposed.

Davis's remarks lead us to reason that individual family members experienced the consequences of a decline in mortality by way of having to live with several siblings with whom they were obliged to share whatever they could obtain from their parents. Several additional implications suggest that the individual family member might have become preoccupied with having to spend more time with his parents because of an economic obligation to help support the family. As an adult, because he had been raised among many siblings, he would have fewer resources with which to start his own family and to provide for educating his own children and endowing their marriages.

Davis addresses the assumption of similar orientations within families in northwest Europe and Japan during the historic periods under review, but he does not deal with the measurement of the orientations and the implied communication involved at the level of social interaction.

Substantive problems having to do with class differences in towns, cities, and agricultural areas (particularly with respect to presumed inheritance troubles described by demographers) are neatly questioned by Davis; who reminds us that individuals and family groups react to changing perceptions and definitions of their socially organized settings rather than responding to "traditional values."

In the case of a rural population's demographic response to declining mortality, Davis tries to pinpoint the critical decisions affecting changes in fertility behavior. Declining mortality leads to land scarcity and changes in traditional patterns of land distribution for couples wanting to get married. Land scarcity problems lead to postponement of marriage and to the migration of rural youth to find nonagricultural jobs created by a changing economy. Davis reasons that the decisions to postpone marriage and leave agriculture were probably made jointly. The actor's commonsense interpretations of his everyday life circumstances remains a tacit but central feature of Davis's description of possible substantive decisions within the family.

Davis implies that members decided to postpone marriage and to leave the farm setting because they saw that this declining mortality (and hence, under the present argument, overpopulation) were contributing to a scarcity of land. The "responses" of postponing marriage and migrating to nonagricultural occupational possibilities are linked to changes in the larger economy, whereby industrialization requires emigration from agricultural areas. The rural youth who moved to the city, which was the locus of industrialization, were "rewarded" for such migration. Farms were supplied with needed capital, farm youth were able to marry, and so on. These activities can be viewed as having provided an "alerted" or self-conscious population with the opportunities to participate in the economic revolution. For these youth, Davis notes, there was no "resistance" to modernization in terms of adhering to a "traditional value system." Thus the rural population of industrialized countries "responded" to declining mortality by out-migration and a postponement of marriage, not simply to reduce fertility or to lessen the population problem, "but as a response to the complexity and insecurity of the new requirements for respectable adult status under changing circumstances" (Davis 1963: 355–356). Thus Davis seems to rely on an implicit model of the actor who makes everyday interpretations to perceived environmental changes. Knowledge of the structure of everyday interaction, therefore, is essential for a viable demographic theory.

Davis emphasizes that conditions external to daily family life, such as knowledge and technology, can influence declining mortality, industrialization, and economic development. His work suggests that the locus of change resides in the day-to-day living patterns and decisions within the nuclear family. Families presumably were faced with recognizing the social significance of declining mortality and the opportunities of a developing society. To maintain their social status and consumption (or perhaps to improve either or both), they had to alter their demographic behavior. The plausible substantive conclusions advanced by Davis, therefore, presuppose an implicit model of the actor and a theory of social organization that makes use of, but does address, the researcher's resources as a member of some group or society. The researcher makes implicit use of his ability as a member to imagine or construct typical courses of action for fellow members, to attribute typical motives, and to assume the existence of practical reasoning to satisfy the observer's thinking about practical action based on his conception of the settings.

Problems of Demographic Analysis.   In this section I discuss some of the issues that are slighted or ignored by the demographer.

The demographer does not question the nature of the demographic stimulus. Is the stimulus intended to alert the reader to a feasible way of "talking about" conditions leading to changes in population size, density, reproduction, and so on? References made by the demographer to "stimulus" conditions occur after the fact; hence the researcher can always claim "responses" while obscuring the nature of the stimuli.

Davis's paper forces us to ask whether persons in everday settings are actually responding to the kinds of stimuli that demographers mention as relevant. For example (to simplify the issue), suppose that people do respond, by migrating and using contraceptives, to a decline in infant mortality and to the observation of a sustained natural increase in population arising from this change in mortality. The presumed reasoning is that some upper bound on the number of children per family is viewed as desirable and thus will be reflected in the everyday and long-range motives of respondents. The demographer assumes that a "realization" occurs that fewer children are dying or that this datum is somehow made relevant to the respondents. The demographer's reasoning implies that there is an "awareness" that a "certain" number of children seem to be dying and that this condition is supposed to lead to the decision to have more or fewer children. If my reasoning is crude, it is partly due to the difficulty of finding in demographers' writings explicit statements about the kinds of activities and reasoning of respondents that are presupposed in the macro statements demographers make.

If we now refer to the population at large rather than to infants only, the general assumptions of the demographer appear to be that members of a group or society link a decline in mortality to a sustained natural increase in population, and that they then "reason" that fewer births are necessary to sustain the desired number of children or to live within the economic level or funds available for the family.

A difficult problem in demographic statements about abstract stimuli and responses is ascertaining how members monitor and evaluate activities associated with changes in population. The demographer evaluates such activities *after the fact*. But how do individual members come to recognize the existence of "high" or "low" mortality, and how is such information transmitted to others? To which others is it transmitted, and with what effects? How do courses of action become identified by the researcher and by the respondent or generalized "member," and how are they then implemented? Are courses of action that reduce births or con ceptions the result of perceived natural increases beyond some limit? The information we might have about such interactional settings is seldom linked to the "objective" tables used by the demographer.

Demographers and sociological population experts have not addressed the questions of how members come to receive, store, ignore, or "misunderstand" information, how they process different types of information that are received, and how they subsequently produce courses of action that are said to reflect "values" or "attitudes." Yet the abstract language used by demographers to describe the population characteristics of a group, sample, nation-state, or culture area, implies tacit understanding of interactional settings. For example, references to personal and national goals are implied in demographic discussions of "responses" to sustained natural increase in population. These abstract references cannot ignore but must reflect members' methods of "knowing," theorizing, and contemplating or taking courses of action in coming to terms with everyday life circumstances.

Studying everyday interactional settings is basic to sociology because members allude to or discuss such subjects as sexual relations, family size, the use of contraceptives, and household movements, during context-sensitive activities. This means that the study of fertility behavior and other demographic concerns should be applications of theories about interactional settings and how members create accounts to represent their everyday experiences.

Let us consider an example of how the demographer reasons "what could have happened": demographic data show that Polish mothers living on farms between 1855 and 1880 had fewer children, irrespective of marital postponement and rural–urban migration, as the size of the farm (in hectares) decreased. The demographer then assumes that a concern with the loss of relative status had its impact despite the "adjustment mechanisms" of marital postponement and migration. This reasoning is suggested directly by the use of tables with arbitrary cutoff points into which data are coded and arranged. The inferences about status and adjustment mechanisms occur in an interactional vacuum. We are not told how to use ethnographic materials about life in rural Poland during the period named. Furthermore, demographers do not make use of extensive ethnographic or sociolinguistic materials now available when they analyze vital statistics and census materials of the twentieth century.

But suppose the abstract notions of relative lack of status and "values" centering around desire for more leisure time, along with religious considerations, are in fact correlated for high or low fertility in different families. I would like to advance the argument that there is little evidence at the level of day-to-day interaction to show how such notions are discussed by family members, or how such discussions, if they take place, are to be located vis-à-vis other activities of the families. Are these notions central or peripheral to the family? Are they discussed frequently or seldom? And when discussed, do they figure prominently in the day-to-day preoccupations of the husband and wife? Are they merely occasional conversational topics that mask concerns about infidelity or other family problems? If these substantive issues are so vital to the demographer's interests, why are they not studied independently of surveys about fertility?

An examination of interviews conducted in this study suggests that fertility issues per se are often irrelevant to many families and their day-to-day problems of living. This does not mean that such issues are never discussed—simply that respondents do not reveal a preoccupation with these topics in their answers to our questions. Our survey questions impose a rigid format on the study of fertility issues. A broader context of family life must be understood if the substantive issue of fertility is of interest to the demographer. When we study fertility in "developed" and "underdeveloped" countries, we must modify our ideal-type conception of the middle-class respondent who aspires for higher status, more leisure, and more material objects.

Fertility rates, therefore, may be only fortuitously connected with the "causal variables" described by demographers. Thus the "causal" nature of such variables may be plausible when examined within the context of the questionnaire's constraints on what members can say to each other (and to researchers) about their activities. The interviews or the questionnaires' accounts about fertility behavior may be independent of the day-to-day activities that produce differentials in the number of live births. The "causal" chain may be an artifact of the verbal accounts of members and the researcher's coding procedures and methods for obtaining data and assembling tables. Accounts by family members indexing fertility issues surely emerge in day-to-day family interaction, but their significance for fertility rates remains a mystery not explored by demographers. Differences in the means by which everyday accounts are produced by members for their own consumption and for the consumption of researchers remains a central sociological concern. How these often different accounts are to be related to the practical problems of fertility control is of applied concern to some sociologists. In this book I suggest an approach for using the study of the structure of everyday interaction and communication to serve both interests.

Concluding Remarks. One major sociological approach to the study of population problems might be termed the "table of organization" view, in which the actor's social position in society is believed to mold his dispositions to behave in predictable ways. Role taking in everyday life is a function of position in the social structure. A recent paper stresses the idea that roles are less-institutionalized statuses. Statuses that are "institutionalized" are based on third-party consensus in the community about norms and values (Goode 1960) . Rewards and punishments are meted out according to a double type of rationality. Activities that contribute most to the society's survival over time are likely to be highly valued. Hence, on the one hand, the performance of activities that are functionally necessary for survival creates a table of organization (or interrelated statuses) that comes to be valued; on the other hand, that which is valued provides an orientation to the actor-members of the society for guiding their conduct and generating abstract rules for ensuring a system of rewards and punishments that contributes to the control of individuals and groups. Everyday communication, ritual activities, and written laws (i.e., "mutual expectations") serve as constant reminders of the values and norms of the society and form a kind of idealized order to which everyone tends to subscribe.

The table of organization view stands in contrast to the cognitive sociological view, which is concerned with everyday social interaction. Thus the cognitive view emphasizes the actor's theories and methods of accounting for and producing the everyday social organization which the sociologist labels the normative structure of society.

In the table of organization theory, societies undergoing economic development are said to pass through a demographic transition whereby high death and birth rates are lowered. The important question is then how quickly the birth rate can be lowered after a fall in the death rate occurs. Some writers (Freedman 1963) assume that a parallel kind of rationality is used in the development of the economic system, on the one hand, and the emergence of an "awareness" in the population regarding the rewards and importance of family planning and lower fertility, on the other. This line of thought implies that "good reasons" exist for families to desire large and then small families. For example, researchers may assume that if males are considered to be important for carrying on existing traditions viewed as valuable to the maintenance of the society, then families will "overproduce" until it becomes possible to demonstrate that a small number of children (which includes males) will survive with improved health conditions. Hence attempts to lower fertility are not to be recommended by the policy planner until death rates have been lowered and general health conditions improved.

This argument is of interest because it links kinship structure with societal values and norms, and with the problems of population growth and economic development. The problems associated with transforming the "developing" or "underdeveloped" areas of the world into industrialized societies, and finding ways to make the lives of people in industrial societies "happier," more "worthwhile," or "richer," are not viewed as conceptual problems of theory—understanding the interface between the actor's situated behavior and his normative perspective—but primarily as "technical" problems that are solvable in "due time."

However, suppose we merely view the family as a semiautonomous system of interaction that is continuously preoccupied with its own problems of remaining viable and of coming to terms with an essentially difficult form of social organization that family members might view as incompatible. From such an approach, general and abstract basic values and norms of the society would be peripheral to an understanding of how families emerge through various marriage situations, how families sustain themselves over time, or how they dissolve and/or become reconstituted in different arrangements. Basic or ideal values may be invoked during interviews by researchers or by the marriage (divorce) partners; but this often serves as a means of rationalizing or normalizing or justifying decisions already taken. Hence values about family size and family planning or about any other facet of societal existence and practice are not very useful if the values are conceived as general and abstract static entities, "internalized" by the actor in the course of socialization. The values and norms are also presumed to be external in the sense that organized rituals, organizations, governmental propaganda, and mass media provide a context within which the actor periodically is reminded and reminds himself of his allegiance to certain valued traditions and practices and beliefs.

Most of the information on fertility and family planning has been acquired by using some variant of social or sample surveys whereby standard questions are asked orally or in written form, and participants select their answers from a set of precoded responses. This methodological strategy is particularly suitable if we accept the rationality of the theory proposed earlier concerning kinship, economic development, population growth, and the survival of society over time. Since the individual responds to a conception of the world within the framework provided by the researcher, his conceptions of himself and of his way of life, too, are researcher-oriented. This circumstance enables the researcher to decide where the individual stands in the general scheme of things, linking kinship with economic development and population growth. This methodology has built into it both abstract theory and substance, and the actor's interview participation remains somewhat passive and divorced from his actual day-to-day activities.

In conclusion, the table of organization view stresses the actor's location in the social order vis-à-vis others—including his familial, occupational, educational, and religious affiliations or experiences, which are all viewed as factors in accounting for the actor's expected behavior.

The alternate perspective proposed here focuses on the actor's lived, everyday experiences (Schutz, 1962, 1964; Garfinkel 1967). The lived experiences are reflected in the actor's use of language categories and nonverbal communication. The communicational skills available to the actor combine with commonsense reasoning to provide him with broad procedures for interpreting everyday experiences. The actor achieves stability in his perception and interpretation of his environment through an interface between cognitive or interpretive procedures and idealized normative rules (Cicourel 1973). The field researcher confronts the same problem. Hence when we as researchers, in seeking to obtain information from subjects, enter into a social relationship of the kind necessary for an interview, and then pose questions, record answers, interpret the answers as a basis for further questions, and the like, we must rely on cognitive or interpretive procedures.

Both observer and respondent employ verbal and nonverbal methods for making the social structures of everyday life observable. The observer's task is complicated by his own implicit use of cognitive processes and commonsense accounts and reasoning for entering the respondent's environment, sustaining the social relationship, posing questions, receiving answers, evaluating the respondent's environment, and interpreting the findings to others. The observer must also weigh the respondent's evaluation of the interviewer, the questions posed, how the answers are formulated—all within the interactional context that operates for the respondent.

The chapters that follow reflect the questions and issues exposed here. I have tried to clarify my concerns with comparative methodological issues and the structure of everyday interaction through a study of Argentine fertility.

CHAPTER 2

Two Views of Decision-Making and
Some Consequences for Field Studies of Fertility

In discussing the substantive areas of reproductive behavior and family organization, researchers refer to the "decisions" that are said to influence family interaction and the social context of reproduction. Social scientists invariably tie decision-making to an implicit or explicit conception of rationality. In this chapter I want first to discuss decision-making in the family, then to deal briefly with the problem of rationality, and finally to ask how we are to clarify family decision-making behavior when the data-gathering procedures used in our field studies are not related to the everyday behavioral environment within which choices are made by members. By critically examining a recent discussion of field studies of fertility and family organization, I seek to clarify some of the theoretical and methodological issues seldom addressed, or treated casually, by workers in the area.

A Contemporary Model of Decision–Making. By referring to decision-making in the family, we imply that partners recognize possible "choices." Choosing from among the various alternatives that are available results in an orientation to and an organization of activities. In looking at the relationship of modern technology to family planning, the researcher often asks, "What values or purposes do partners seek to satisfy through adoption of family planning practices?" Some assume that the mere availability of family planning practices (or technology) is an insufficient explanation for its use. Recent works stress husband–wife interaction—noting, for example, that the effectiveness of contraceptives requires cooperation between partners, or that routinized behavior patterns are linked to strong motivation to continue use of contraceptives (Stycos 1955; Hill, Stycos, and Back 1959; Rainwater 1960; Blake 1961; Stycos and Back 1964; Rainwater 1965). Cooperation and the use of contraceptives means that a couple must maintain a high level of self-control. Nevertheless, researchers continue to discuss the socially organized context of bounded family encounters without clear statements about everyday rationality and about basic issues of organized social life. Abstract generalizations are common—for example, that the demographic transition can be attributed to the diffusion of technology throughout society (Beshers 1967: 69).

Beshers's recent work (1967: Chapters 3 and 4), however, provides a valuable guide to the possible use of decision theory in conceptualizing fertility behavior within a family. Beshers's formulation and the perspective used in my study furnish background for understanding the analysis of data in subsequent chapters. I begin by summarizing Beshers's use of decision theory to characterize how hypothetical individuals produce behavioral outcomes described as communication patterns and as relationships within a group.

1. Each hypothetical individual or actor is seen to have characteristic attributes such as age, sex, and experiences based on participation in some organized setting ("society"). The actor has had historical exposure to various events such as wars and economic depressions, which contribute to the society's history and to the actor's recognition of and orientation toward his environment.

2. The actor selects decisions from among a specifiable set of available alternatives. The alternatives and criteria used by the actor in his or her selection are specifiable by the researcher's theory and form the basis for describing the actor's perspective.

3. The actor's selections are assumed to be motivated by the different consequences he or she attributes to each of the alternatives. However, no attempt is made to assess the "conscious content of the individual's mind" (Beshers 1967: 77) when the selection behavior occurs.

4. It is assumed that the actor has partial perception of the alternatives and their consequences but that variations exist in the alternatives perceived across a given population. Different selective processes are used by the various members of a population. Beshers notes that the classical economic description of the decision-making problem makes different assumptions: (a) the decision-maker knows all the possible alternatives and can provide each alternative with a pair of numbers, (b) one number stands for the *"likelihood of the alternative"* or the probability that it will

occur, (c) the other number stands for the "*utility of alternative*" or its desirability by the actor, and (d) the actor can use the product of the pair of numbers as an index for each alternative to compare various alternatives vis-à-vis the maximum utility he might expect them to yield.

5. In Beshers's explanation (1967:78) of the decision-making activity, the decision process changes over time for the actor (as opposed to the rather static conception of maximizing or minimizing risk in decision-making in classical theorizing). Hence Beshers's point that changes may occur over time leads to a notion of sequential decision-making.

6. The sequential reestimating of the utility of various alternatives and their probabilities over time suggests the idea of different, emergent decision rules that require the decision-maker to make use of new information from the environment.

7. The actor's receipt of new information directs the researcher's attention to the actor's conception about the value of long- and short-run rewards and his comparison of such rewards. From this information the investigator predicts the actor's choice.

8. Beshers's model appears to define the set of alternatives available to the actor and their relevant possibilities, including the actor's unawareness of alternatives. Beshers (1967: 80), however, notes that such a procedure does not enable the investigator to distinguish between the actor's ignorance of an alternative and the researcher's estimation that the alternative has a likelihood of zero.

9. The actor's use of a decision rule is always embedded within his emotional structure, which is influenced by the kinds of close personal relationships established from childhood on. Thus his utilities are resistant to change and are rooted in a kind of emotional bedrock. The actor's attitudes are said to reflect the stability of utilities. The actor who is instrumentally oriented therefore, would, rely less on his emotional attachments and more on new information as articulated with his cognitive expectations of the likelihood of alternatives. Conversely, if an actor's accounting system is oriented by his emotional structure, new information would be ignored.

10. An actor's close personal relationships become key elements in predicting his utility structure, hence the kind of orientation he would have toward decisions. Moreover, the actor's close personal relationships are linked directly to marriage and kinship relationships, particularly insofar as such relationships include communication patterns pertaining to values about fertility behavior. Thus the model directs attention to abstract values derived from kinship relationships.

11. Two methodological consequences of the theoretical decision-making model are (a) attitudinal items in questionnaires can be used to ask subjects about values, and (b) the behavioral consequences of imputed values (based on the researcher's estimates) can be deduced to check the values against correlates from census and vital statistics data. Specifying the characteristics of the husband and the wife would lead to statements about their relationship and about the values subscribed to by each (Beshers 1967: 83) .

12. Societies can be characterized as "traditional" or "modern," and the researcher is interested in changes from one state of the society to another. He also wants to know how a "breakdown" in the former state leads to changes in how actors make decisions. Beshers (1967: 85) uses three "modes of orientation" to depict the actor's decision-making—"traditional," "short-run hedonistic," and "purposive-rational."

13. The actor operating with a traditional mode of orientation bases all his decisions on what has always been the case in his culture; hence new information is irrelevant (or not recognized as "new?"). No future time perspective exists. The prediction of the actor's behavior is said to be based on a knowledge of his society's "customs and culture," and not on a knowledge of his own "psychological characteristics."

14. The short-run hedonistic mode orients the actor to likelihoods and utilities that extend into a brief future period. "Evanescent situational factors" are presumed to be the relevant conditions for predicting the actor's behavior, and, therefore, the actor's "immediate psychological situation" influences his or her decision-making.

15. The purposive-rational mode is the orientation attributed to an actor who possesses a time perspective that extends into some indefinite future and who is capable of calculating complex likelihoods and utilities New information becomes a critical resource for this actor in making sequential decisions.

The general threads running through the foregoing provide a clear means of understanding how the model would be applied hypothetically to fertility behavior. Each mode of orientation indexes our expectations of how a given actor will define his or her situation, recognize and utilize new information, interact with the sanctions of the society, adopt innovative family planning activities, and so on.

Beshers (1967: 87) specifies the emergence of actor types by using the Weberian notion of rationality and an abstract historical account of the modification of Western feudal society. The consistency of the model, however, is not to be found in a behavioral sociolinguistic environment.

Besher's theory does not link the means used by actors to sustain social organization vis-à-vis some conception, use, and articulation of norms and values to the means by which they generate courses of action deemed "acceptable" to others through recognition, orientation, and organization of their perception and understanding of actual settings. Day-to-day social interaction is depicted (hence truncated) by a conceptual schema in which everyday behavior becomes relevant only when *compressed into packaged atemporal episodes,* called answers to questions, and used to obtain census or questionnaire materials.

The theory presented by Beshers is valuable because it makes explicit assumptions that are usually tacit or ignored as irrelevant in sociological and demographic research on the family and fertility behavior. My criticisms would be difficult to formulate without Beshers's statement. Thus I propose a competing framework rather than merely rejecting the view proposed by Beshers.

A limitation of attitude-type or census studies is their reliance on information divorced from the interview settings and the day-to-day action scenes of those whose activities are being described and analyzed. Any theory we employ must utilize procedures for making sense of every-day interaction as well as the exchanges produced by structured elicitation procedures. We need to learn how members routinely question one another, and we must contrast such informal questioning with our knowledge of how structured questions produce information.

I make no claims here to a general theory of interrogation. I merely indicate a few possible approaches to resolving some of the problems encountered in dealing with data that are reconstructed (in unknown ways) from everyday conversational and nonverbal activities. These brief remarks, combined with a discussion of the problem of rationality, are used to develop a model to contrast with Beshers's model. In the present study I tried to satisfy the following assumptions and methodological conditions.

If we can pose question in a general but often purposely ambiguous way, permitting the respondent to recognize them as relevant to his particular circumstances, the subject's response should encode elements of his original experiences. These elements are made known by his use of intonation, his choice of lexical items and their syntactic structure, and by the kinds of socially relevant categories he employs. (A fixed-choice item, with its highly restricted set of alternatives, may never capture the subject's range of everyday experiences and the spontaneous categories expected from a cross section of some population. Nor would a pretested interview schedule help provide more "appropriate" categories for the subject to use in formulating his response. The respondent must be allowed spontaneous expression, free from the researcher's restrictive questions.)

The subject's response always stands as an index of wider meanings, which the researcher must elaborate with his theory. Traditional data-reduction coding of responses formally eliminates this wider context of meanings packed into the categories employed by the researcher to capture the respondent's experiences. The researcher who makes traditional explanations after the tables are assembled uses his tacit inferences about the meaning of the original questions and answers as a *hidden resource.* These inferences are later incorporated into his theory and interpretations to the reader. Thus the researcher expects the tables to "speak for themselves." His analysis, however, relies on his commonsense interpretation of the original questions and answers and the tables.

My present perspective directs the researcher's attention to the member's situated use of commonsense reasoning (Schutz 1964; Garfinkel 1967). This reasoning is tied to settings and consists of *interpretive procedures* (Cicourel 1973) that give the member a sense of social structure. The interpretive procedures enable the researcher and the member to *recognize* "appropriate" settings, talk, and activities, thus providing an *orientation* to their environment. The interpretive procedures enable both researcher and member to *organize* relevant interpretations about what is "happening" and about what courses of action should be pursued.

The interpretive procedures of the researcher and the respondent are like tacit instructions to examine the "appropriate" or "normal" forms of social structure presumably communicated by a question, and the corresponding social structure revealed in an answer. What implied information does the question-answer pair contain that may or may not be indexed by a category or phrase in the dialogue exchanged by interviewer and respondent? The researcher uses this implied information to elaborate on the data obtained by an explicit elicitation procedure.

As a conversation continues, the participants (interviewer and interviewee) rely on *reflexive* thinking about the talk itself and the material discussed, and about the relevance of each one's biography, the setting of the interview, and the impact that each participant has on the other one owing to their respective appearances and self-presentations. Because of this reflexiveness, interpretations that are placed on initial questions and answers later become integral features in each participant's gradual

assumption that he "knows" the other. Thus later questions and answers take on added meanings by virtue of previous interpretations.
The label "rapport" is not adequate here because it masks the activities
whereby the ongoing interaction acquires context-restricted meanings
that are not specified or intended by the questionnaire or interview items.
My view contrasts with Beshers's model by stressing that the methodological strategy as an information-processing system creates the data in
ways that are not examined in conjunction with emergent interpretations.
Hence Beshers's reference to the likelihood and utility of an alternative
is an emergent feature of the interactional setting that trades on a larger
stored data base.

We search the original questions and answers for categories that would
signal unstated or implied information indexing member-organized relationships and reasoning. The categories index relationships between persons and activities formed by socially prescribed rules. The categories,
and their larger collectional or componential basis, are linked to persons
by contrasting information assumed to be integral to the members'
socially distributed and socially sanctioned knowledge (Goodenough
1957; Frake 1962; Sacks 1967). When the researcher locates a category in
a larger frame or collection (age, sex, kinship), he presumes knowledge
of how members situationally select appropriate categories for expressing
their experiences and knowledge about social organization.

The question–answer format presumes that the participants know how
to recognize "appropriate" questions and answers, that they know when
someone has terminated a question–answer unit, and that they know the
"rights" of each participant regarding who is to speak or listen. A practical problem here has to do with the researcher's ability to recognize
and organize probing, to decide whether he has received an appropriate
answer, or to feel that a question may be inappropriate.

The foregoing remarks are theoretically oriented methodological strategies and presuppositions necessary for guiding the development of a
decision-making model involving both the actor *and* the researcher.

The Problem of Rationality. The three ideal-typical modes of orientation
described by Beshers are consistent with the static notion that "attitudes
and values" are possessed by the actor and are inculcated throughout
childhood in an unspecified manner. The actor somehow acquires characteristics that are the product of his culture and thus he becomes
traditionally oriented. Or the actor is oriented to action vis-à-vis the
"immediate psychological situation." Or finally, the actor is capable of

processing new information in such a way that he entertains an extended time perspective and makes the best use of present and past experiences. The key or pivotal element in Beshers's formulation is the extent to which the actor's emotional structure affects his use of new information in conjunction with past and future relationships (the question of recognition of new information is not problematic for Beshers). Three factors are important here: (1) stable or unstable attitudes and values as established or anchored in early experiences, (2) the influence of the actor's emotional structure on the processing of new information, and (3) the interpretations placed on concrete or hypothetical action scenes by the actor. The researcher's model does not reveal the *interactions* among these factors, nor does the model specify how questionnaire items or census or vital statistics materials would reveal (much less include) the elements of the model said to produce decisions.

There is no theory of data to show how actors or members encode verbal and nonverbal behavior by processing the internal and external stimuli experienced by them. Such a theory might enable us to examine systematically the elements of Beshers's model and the structure of inter- action that produces decisions. Without a theory of data, questions and answers are presumed to possess "obvious" significance. Furthermore, lacking a theory of data, the researcher declines to ascertain how the questions posed are attended to by respondents with the result that their answers both fit within the specifiable alternatives envisaged by the researcher and, at the same time, presumably encode unique experiences that faithfully index action scenes or observations the subject has en- countered.

The types of "rationality" contained in Beshers's modes of orientation cluster around one of several types of actor—one who is more or less "programmed" by ideal normative customs, one who is responsive to context-restricted conditions, or one who can weigh competing (old and new) information and establish complex likelihoods and utilities. Thus the first type of actor would not recognize situational factors as relevant or would be indifferent to them, whereas the second type would be responsive only to situated circumstances, and the third type, by striking a balance between the first two types, would be capable of rational planning. The actor's cognitive structure is depicted as static in the traditional mode of orientation, capricious in the short-run hedonistic mode, and optimally "rational" or "sensible" in the purposive-rational mode.

The traditional mode presupposes that the researcher can lay out an ideal normative theory of culture to which the actor is automatically responsive; the actor either recognizes "appropriate" stimuli and ignores "unacceptable" messages, or he compensates for noise in the channel and somehow "normalizes" discrepant scenes. The researcher's task appears to be simple—show how such an actor's mode of orientation articulates with his mannner of making choices in everyday life. *How* he chooses is never clear when the respondent is only given fixed-choice questionnaire items that restrict selections to precoded alternatives. These items only permit the emergence of the researcher's conception of likely alternatives, which conveniently correspond to the three hypothetical modes of orientation. In Beshers's model, the process whereby choices are recognized by the actor as relevant and are negotiated is never examined.

In conventional theories of rationality, everyday organizational behavior by actors is depicted as rational when appropriate means for the attainment of ends are based on factual rather than value premises and are selected within a clearly specified hierarchy of organization (Blau and Scott 1962). How actors decide on what is "appropriate" remains an untouched empirical issue.

According to the view (Schutz 1943) of rationality I follow in this book, the appropriateness of a means for realizing an intended end is not simply a matter of presumably clear organizational objectives (in the present case, familial objectives). Rather, the perception of means and objectives must be understood as a process that is relative to the actor's typified conceptions of practical adequacy. Whatever is "rational" about administrative activities, law statutes, household budgeting, or fertility behavior, always occurs in the context of everyday experience and typifications based on past conduct.

Schutz suggests that the actor makes sense of his environment by creating loose equivalence classes (as opposed to clear-cut true–false categories). The typifications in the actor's stock of knowledge interacts with emergent meanings from a setting to concretize what is likely or unlikely. When the actor concretizes an ambiguously defined scene, he creates a temporally bounded set by experiential fiat, thus achieving practical decision-making. The practical rationality exhibited by the actor is an emergent phenomenon and is not directed by fixed modes of orientation; instead, the actor invokes rules in creating accounts of "what happened."

Issues in Field Studies of Fertility.   Beshers stresses (*a*) the actor's mode of orientation in assessing and acting on long-range consequences, (*b*) the purposive-rational actor's "calculation of the future status of children" when planned births are linked to budget considerations, and (*c*) the decision processes used by couples in trying to coordinate selection of goals with types of birth control methods.

In examining the results of the pioneering Indianapolis study (1958) of fertility, Beshers finds support for his model [and discusses the model by reference to Weber (1947) and Banks (1954)] in the investigators' claims that social class is negatively correlated with family size and that for families who planned all births there is a positive correlation between number of children and economic position. Beshers believes that the validity of his model is further substantiated by the findings that planning decreases as we move from salaried professionals to lower income occupations, and that fertility behavior is adjusted to fit the constraints of income to maximize opportunities for children. Still another claim of support for the model is the evidence that fertility is negatively correlated with economic insecurity for those who planned all births. But those families in the total sample who were economically insecure did not plan.

I shall not attempt to summarize all the results of the Indianapolis study, having noted that Beshers finds strong support in this research for his model. Two additional sources of support are the disclosures that (1) a diffusion of the "compulsive personality type" is associated with the purposive-rational mode of orientation, downward from families with high socioeconomic status to lower statuses, and (2) fertility planning can be viewed as a function of "the family as a two-person decision unit."

Beshers seeks further evidence for his theory in the work on Puerto Rico by Hill, Stycos, and Back (1959), which reports a lack of planning on the part of the respondents, as would be expected because of the low-income sample selected. The net result would be a lack of planning, little or no birth control practices before the third pregnancy, and a discrepancy between actual family size and preferred size.

When Beshers reports findings that link "communication" between spouses to planning and marital adjustment, we learn that the respondent was provided with a basis for identifying with an ideal normative conception of Western marriage as promoted in the community or suggested as "correct" by the questionnaire or interview schedule. The researcher does not investigate the members' conceptions of "communication" and "marital adjustment" in terms of the members' accounts of how these notions are produced by their daily activities; rather, he assumes that these concepts are understood in terms of his own restricted questionnaire constructions, which use ambiguous everyday categories. Thus little or no attention is given to the words a member might employ to express such notions to other members, or to the range or kinds of behavior activities such categories as "communication" and "marital adjustment" might subsume for speaker-hearers.

Studies in the United States have led to the following notions about fertility behavior and about other substantive issues of interest to sociologists:

1. Weber's postulate of the "rationalization of society" is taken to mean that the shift from a rural-agrarian to an urban-industrial society is somehow reflected in the actor's modes of orientation to his environment.

2. Egalitarian relations between the sexes as indexed by the rising status of women, women's participation in the labor force, "the middle-class life style," joint decision-making, and the like, have been attributed to the sociologist's prototypical respondent. The sociologist counts on an unexplicated notion of an ideal-typical family to provide him with data that support a progressive disenchantment with traditional activities.

3. This college-educated, upper-middle-class, ideal-typical couple is easily "observed" wherever "modernization" is firmly established or emerging. The social scientist has only to examine his own family to verify his theory. Thus when Freedman, Whelpton, and Campbell (1959: Chapter 4) found that 25% of the college-educated couples in their fertility study had offspring that were not planned, these "mistakes" were not viewed as "deviant cases" that should warrant further study using *different* theoretical suppositions.

4. There is a tacit assumption among researchers that the practical problem of population growth and stability will become steadily "better" as our prototypical upper-middle-income family becomes the dominant or most common urban dweller. In what year will this occur? Some are probably willing to give estimates, but whether such a type will predominate—much less remain in the same ideal-typical arrangement now described in abstract terms—is not at all clear.

5. Because of the much-cherished American notion that some form of therapy (sensitivity training, group, or private) will usually "work things out" for the "better," the ideal-typical family would be expected to maintain "good" communication channels and a "high" level of marital adjustment. This would mean that "rational" behavior can be the only "sensible" outcome.

6. Thus field workers in their own countries or abroad always have a ready-made model for comparative purposes—their own family. A planned

parenthood program would reflect the researcher's family situation to implement the "best" features assumed to be relevant for birth control.

Thus it is clear that researchers can no longer claim present-day America as a guide. We need a comparative perspective that reflects different forms of social organization.

Conclusion. The major conditions leading to differential fertility in Beshers's model are: (*a*) the modes of orientation and their relative frequency in a given population, (*b*) the structural constraint of living in a rural or urban area, (*c*) the channels of personal communication with members of a community, (*d*) the diffusion of information relevant to knowledge about matters such as birth control techniques, (*e*) values about family size as they cross-cut (*a*) and (*b*), and (*f*) the family as a two-person decision process. Other "variables," such as religion, occupation, and communication processes between husband and wife on sex and contraceptives, are also cited by researchers of fertility.

A number of problems not addressed by classical demographic studies are rooted in the field conditions of everyday family life. Anthropologists have shown how "fictionalized" lineage systems (Fallars 1965) have influenced descriptions of ideal kinship formations. Studies of North American and South American families have confounded the status of the ideal-typical family because of the high incidence of divorces at all levels of income and education. The "variables" described in the last paragraph do not take their relevance from a background of carefully described historical and contemporary ethnographic conditions; rather, they rely on the much-used phrase or tacit assumption that "other things are equal" or irrelevant to the operation of these "variables."

Family organization does not necessarily revolve around planning of children or their future, based on such factors as present and future expected income, husband–wife communication about family planning, knowledge about contraceptives, occupation, or rural or urban residence. In sociology, as in demographic studies of family life and fertility behavior, we have yet to clarify the nature of the routine social encounters and the practical decision-making that produce activities we subsume under the label "the family" or "the nuclear family." We have taken over lay definitions and conceptions of family life without bothering to study members's categories for describing familial activities, relationships, and "facts"—these categories are problematic phenomena to be investigated in their own right.

CHAPTER 3

NOTES ON THE ARGENTINE HISTORICAL CONTEXT AND
SOME ETHNOGRAPHIC IMPRESSIONS OF BUENOS AIRES

An Overview of the Argentine Historical Context. It is difficult to
write about a foreign country for an audience which may have only
vague, stereotyped ideas on the subject. For example, the reader may
assume that Argentina is just one more Latin American country,
hence similar to other countries that have been visited or researched or
studied by way of secondary sources. Yet the author has to assume that
the reader knows a bit about the country, then attempt to focus on those
features presumed to be of interest to the reader, for whom the book is
written. In this chapter I have tried to follow a mixed strategy: I cite
works of such authors as Germani (1962, 1965), Romero (1959), Scobie
(1964), and particularly Di Tella, Germani, Graciarena, et al. (1965),
and I use brief descriptions of my own experiences in Buenos Aires and
in a few areas in the Argentine interior. All the authors just named
presume that the reader knows something about the country. Occasionally
I try to balance the problem of citing works by Argentines, which requires
considerable background knowledge for adequate understanding, with
accounts of how I decided I knew something about the country and
about Buenos Aires in particular. I believe this strategy will help to
clarify my attempts at comparative research.

An old problem for which there are few helpful discussions is arriving
at proper descriptions (or appreciating the descriptions of others) when
we have no explicit guidelines for translating experience encoded into
one language and expressed in a second. Since each description is translated by and relies on the background knowledge of the first-language
observer—hence on information not accessible to the second-language
reader—the reader must supply various meanings based on his own

27

notions of what is intended. Thus when I write of my Argentine experiences in American English, I allow the reader to assume that I was oriented to cultural conceptions comparable to the perspectives of an Argentine native speaker. The objectives and experiences described, however, may have been encountered first by me as a tourist-oriented American researcher and transformed because of experiences I had later, when I began to feel I "knew the country better."

I begin with a brief picture of Argentine history as generally presented in the literature. Next, to underscore some problematic features of historical construction which occur when implicit theories are used, I suggest some views that are not entirely consistent with those of the prominent scholars cited. For example, it is easy to attribute such terms as "democracy" or "mass society" to stages in a particular group's development, but it is difficult to show how such conditions came about at the level of day-to-day social interaction. A theory of historical change, like a theory of language change and reconstruction, requires a conception of everyday social organization which includes members' theories and methods for understanding and producing everyday activities. Only with such a framework can historical change be understood and described by the researcher. This description cannot be accomplished unless the researcher's theory and method can address the structure of social interaction depicted by the language used by members studied and the language used by researchers. The language used is often a tacit index of change and stability in social organization. The following historical résumé and ethnographic account is sharply telescoped to provide the reader with a minimal amount of information with which to place in perspective subsequent materials obtained through the use of an interview schedule.

Stages in Argentina's Development.   Scobie (1964) refers to the period 1516–1600 as the discovery and conquest stage of Argentine development. Settlements were established in Buenos Aires (east), Mendoza (west), Tucumán (north), and Córdoba (central), which continue to be centers of population.

In the period 1600–1810, described as the colonial stage, the area now called Argentina consisted of fragmented outposts of the Spanish empire. The development of Buenos Aires, for political and economic reasons, led to a centralized colonial authority that was to be important in movements toward independence. Scobie states that neither dissatisfaction with the system of collecting taxes, nor disenfranchisement, nor friction between Creole and Spanish merchants led to disloyalty or demands for independence, but when Napolean overthrew the Spanish monarchy in 1807-1808, the Creoles of Buenos Aires launched activities (e.g., seeking local government control and opening Buenos Aires to world trade) that eventually resulted in independence. However, the colony, with its predominantly rural population, its urban trade centers, and its considerable centralization at Buenos Aires, was not an organized entity ready to assume independence as a country.

Despite independence from Spain (declared in 1816), there was no central government of Argentina, and a centralist constitution was rejected by the provinces. After a civil war during 1828–1829, the dictatorship of Juan Manuel de Rosas provided autocratic unification for coastal areas, but open rebellion against de Rosas in 1851 ended in his defeat the following year. The period of the colonial regime until 1852 has been called a stage in which a traditional society existed governed by a "boss" or *patron,* whose benevolence could not be taken for granted. This was a period of domination over the rank and file by appointed authorities. An off-and-on civil war between the province of Buenos Aires and the other provinces (1852–1861) continued to preclude integration of the country. From 1862 to 1880 continued consolidation occurred, insurrections were repressed, Indian opposition was eliminated, immigration increased, railroad building emerged, and economic advances were made, culminating in the creation of a federal capital at Buenos Aires and a unified oligarchy under Julio Roca.

Students of Argentine history often refer to 1880 as the turning point in the development of present-day Argentina. It is difficult to evaluate the implications attributed by various authors to the influence of the oligarchy that began in the 1880s, to the impact of massive immigration of Europeans, to the development of political parties, and the like, but such historical milestones represent elements that could plausibly be used to explain current issues. The problem is that all the factors seem or can be made to seem relevant. As with any construction using highly absorbent structural concepts and data, however, any number of allegations or constructions are possible once there is agreement among several scholars that a few factors (e.g., massive immigration, the growth of political parties, and agricultural development) have been identified as having factual and causal status.

The number of plausible constructions of how the past has influenced the present in the case of Argentina is complicated by the views that the country represents something of an enigma. It possesses many of the features that warrant the use of the term "modern," but even though Argentina has been launched economically and has sustained some ongoing development, the country has never been able to progress very far above its initial level. Thus it seems inappropriate to call Argentina "underdeveloped," but using the language of economic development theories is equally unsuitable precisely because official records show no neat pattern of economic growth.

THE OLIGARCHY.   An elite group called the "Generation of the '80s" dominated Argentine political life from the 1880s until the emergence of suffrage in 1912 and the election of Yrigoyen in 1916. Germani (1962) describes this oligarchy as a conservative-liberal group which generated political stability and encouraged immigration, agricultural development, industrialization, and public works—in short, the oligarchy fostered many of the processes for which the label "modernization" has been used.

Laws were passed to promote greater equity in the distribution of land (Cornblit, Gallo, and O'Connell 1965). These laws, passed in 1864, 1876, 1882, and 1884, were analogous to the Land Acts passed in the United States, but the net result fell far short of the legislative goals. According to Cornblit, Gallo, and O'Connell, there tended to be more concentration of land in fewer hands, because the practical implementation of the laws only served to enhance processes of control by a few groups which the legislation sought to combat.

The above mentioned authors, using descriptive statistical materials and quotations from political speeches, congressional speeches, presidential messages, correspondence, and newspaper accounts, attempt to document the major sources of Argentine immigration from southern Europe. The impact of this massive immigration on Argentina's growth is stated first in terms of sheer numbers (Germani 1962: 185): in 1914 the foreign-born in Argentina formed a little more than 30% of the population (2,389,155 in the total population of 7,885,000). By comparison, the percentage of foreign-born in the United States in 1910 was 14.4. By 1930 Argentina had absorbed some 6,405,000 immigrants, and her population had reached 11,746,000 (Germani 1962: 185), and the United States had admitted some 32,244,000 immigrants and had reached a total population of a little more than 100 million. Much has been said about the social and political impact of the great waves of immigration on Argentina's small population base (Germani 1962: 197–216). Cornblit, Gallo, and O'Connell (1965: 29) suggest that initially there was poor integration of the immigrants into Argentina's political life. These authors state that the immigrants were not very interested in becoming assimilated because of their lack of political participation in the countries of southern Europe from which they came. Evidence for a lack of "commitment" to political participation is said to be found in the tendency for many Italian immigrants (in Argentina, Brazil, and the United States) to return to their native land.

Authors comment on the apparent "looseness" of the political "commitment," the ambiguous system of naturalization throughout the Americas, and the frequent occasions on which Argentine legislation favored foreign-born residents who were not naturalized but who still enjoyed the protection of their country of origin. Finally, the various writers on Argentina note that the existing political structure of the country did not encourage or permit political participation. This ban on participation is often cited as the basis for the immigrants' indifference to elections—an indifference that is said to have already existed among native-born Argentines.

An idea of the distinctiveness of Argentine immigration comes from Germani (1962: 184), who cited the distribution of different European groups for the period 1857-1958: Italian descent, 46%; Spanish descent, 33%; and others, 21%. The "other" category includes Poles, Germans, eastern European Jews, French, English (or Irish or Welsh), Swiss, and persons of Scandinavian or Arabic background.

The Demographic picture is carefully documented by Germani. He explains the significance of these data with plausible, consistent comments which are in accordance with structural-functional American sociological writings about the emergence of urbanized Western countries. Germani describes Argentina's transition from a "traditional" society—based on southern European immigrants' cultural traits, such as attitudes toward politics, family life, work, agriculture, and saving money, and aspirations toward social betterment—to the development of a "mass" society. Argentina lacked a rapidly growing industrial network, a westward land expansion movement, and the puritanical work ethic attributed to the United States. Instead, Argentina is viewed as a country in which land development was less than adequate and industrialization weak, neither being accompanied by the type of immigration that could support the development of agriculture and industry. There were no existing institutions for political development, and the electorate was impoverished and unsophisticated.

The amount of early foreign capital development invested in the country was high. During the Generation of the '80s foreign (primarily British) capital had control of 10 to 15% of the national wealth (Cornblit, Gallo, O'Connell 1965: 35; Conde: Chapter 3.)

The problem of foreign investment evolved into a political issue that even now dominates national political campaigns. Di Tella and Zymelman (1965: Chapter 6) describe six stages in Argentina's economic history: (1) the "traditional" period up to 1853; (2) the period of transition between 1853 and 1880; (3) the period from 1880 to 1914, in which the preconditions of economic development were established; (4) the stage from 1914 to 1933, called the "Big Delay," which was marked by less foreign investment (because of World War I) rather than by the expected economic takeoff; (5) the "takeoff" stage of some industrialization, from 1933 to 1952; (6) and the period from 1952 to the present, which is called the stage of readjustment. Since 1952, Argentina has maintained a status quo in economic development—once more, rather than "taking off" dramatically, as expected. This is attributed to the negative interaction between an unstable political situation and ambivalent governmental policies toward foreign investments and outside aid. The negative interaction has been worsened because foreign countries have developed cautious policies toward Argentina's so-called good or bad climates of investment or aid.

The description of Argentina during its stages of demographic and economic transformation is also said to be mirrored in the country's political development. A central element in Argentina's political development was the emergence of the Radical Civic Union party (Unión Cívica Radical) during the reign of the "conservative-liberal" oligarchy of the 1880s. Around 1891 this party called for political reforms and universal male suffrage, gaining the support of the growing middle classes (Scobie: 1964; Gallo and Sigal: 1965). According to Gallo and Sigal (1965: 134–135), the radical party was primarily a force dedicated to political reform and male suffrage, but it had little or no common front or program on social and economic problems.

With the election of Roque Saenz Peña to the presidency in 1910 there was a shift in the oligarchy, with Saenz Peña leading the way to the right to vote for males in 1912. In the next election (1916) Hipolito Yrigoyen was elected the first radical president. (The term "radical" in the Argentine context refers to middle-of-the-road voters.) The election of Yrigoyen presumably meant that the middle classes had a larger voice in running the country. It is difficult to find descriptive, much less analytic, statements permiting more specific inferences on the subject of how various Argentines felt at the time about the different political changes just described. More than a few writers feel that Argentine political changes were irrelevant to many residents because of a lack of identification with their new country, the attraction of the old, and the obstacles to full participation that Argentine political life placed before both natives and immigrants.

By the time the political changes described had occurred, the country had long established a basic division among the overpowering federal capital of Buenos Aires, the heavily populated and rich area known as the "Litoral," which includes the economically most important provinces, and the regions (e.g., Catamarca, La Rioja, Santiago del Estero) that to this day remain "backward" in the eyes of Argentines.

Thus we see that various authors on Argentine history have implied or stated that by the time universal male suffrage arrived, the country had become rather rigid in its internal economic and political development, and that the major industrial and social changes had produced a small upper-class elite, large middle- and working-class groups, and a relatively small poverty-ridden group to be found primarily in the "backward" provinces.

THE MODERN OR CONTEMPORARY PERIOD. To convey the largest amount of information in the shortest space, I shall make several summary statements designed to cover the "modern" period, which is arbitrarily designated as beginning with the Radical party administration of Yrigoyen.

1. The Radicals altered Argentine politics by reinforcing the party apparatus; thereafter patronage was based on loyalty to the party, rather than on achievement. The tactics of the party led to a reliance on (thus enhancement of) the military to quell disturbances and to protect the party in power. Rather than promoting democratic ideals and practices, the Radicals substituted another, not necessarily more efficient, bureaucratic and administrative machinery for the previous oligarchic system (Scobie 1964: 204).

2. The Radicals apparently were unable to carry out reforms that would satisfy the lower and middle classes which had contributed to their victory. Since the interior provinces remained under conservative control, Yrigoyen could not count on congressional support from these areas for changes. Nor could he count on complete party support because of internal strife (Scobie 1964: 205).

3. With the help of the military, the Radicals crushed worker riots in

January 1919, while reforms designed to help the working class (e.g., social security and minimum wage laws) were defeated. Programs intended to further economic development failed. The only success was the university reform of 1918 that began in Córdoba and led to autonomous university government. This could be described as the beginning of a more intensive politicization of university life in Argentina and elsewhere in Latin America (Scobie 1964: 206).

4. In 1922 the Radicals elected another president, Marcelo T. de Alvear, a member of the conservative wing of the party. The next few years were marked by relative prosperity, but there were no significant political innovations. The new president was thought to be closer to the conservatives and the military than to most members of his own party.

5. Agricultural production and exportation, which had begun to increase significantly in 1862 and had continued to show enormous gains because of immigration to the Pampas, were slowed down by 1930, as were the expansion of railroad lines and the demand for agricultural products on the world market. Economic deterioration became serious. In 1930, two years after the reelection of Yrigoyen, the army entered the scene and began a takeover that was to be repeated many times in subsequent years (Ferrer 1963: 106–116). The year 1929 marked the end of a period of rich agricultural expansion in Argentina, and all over the world.

6. The military takeover of 1930 revealed collusion between the conservatives and the military, and, as many authors like to point out, exposed the military's pretense to having a high, if not the highest, responsibility to "protect" the country in times of crisis. The coup was significant because the decision that the time was appropriate seemingly came from and was organized within the military, and the presumed grounds for taking action was a notion of the "destiny" of the military. There never was and probably never will be policy agreement among the different military branches. It is the presumed independence of the military from civil, and especially grass roots support, which is significant when we describe the role of political parties in Argentina. Paradoxically, various authors report that the military takeover enjoyed the support of many civilian groups, members of the Radical party included. The same kind of support was reported by the news media and to me by personal acquaintances in Argentina after the military coup of June 1966. It would appear that politicians and the general population have come to depend on the military to change deteriorating political and economic conditions. What is not clear is how we could assess this apparent civilian

consensus about military takeovers and the consistency of this view over time. We do not know whether the civilian support is short-range or long-range.

7. A military takeover is followed eventually by new elections, as in 1932 when the conservatives took over and governed until 1943. The 1930 takeover is often described as a turning point in the military's conception of rule by civilians. In Argentina, apparently, the military assumed virtual political autonomy and became protective of this autonomy and missionary in its belief that officers possessed the ability to control and govern the country, particularly when any type of national crisis emerged. During different military periods of government, differences among and within various branches of service have made governing Argentina a highly restricted activity, limited to an army, navy, and air force mixed-membership military "club." We know very little, however, about the nature of military allegiances, differences in ideology, or social, economic, and political ties with nonmilitary groups (Scobie 1964: 217–218).

8. The military takeover of 1943 occurred after a period of economic recovery and was linked in many ways to the international politics of World War II, especially to the rise of fascism in Germany and Italy. An organized group of colonels emerged. The political scene became rather complicated because of the climb to power of Juan D. Perón, who occupied important positions in the new military government, among them Minister of War and the new post of Labor Secretary. Perón supported labor groups, who began to hear that he was offering unheard-of governmental support for working-class problems. In 1944 Perón was made vice president of the country, and according to an informant whom I knew well from a small study of a textile union local, Perón sent organizers to working-class suburbs of Buenos Aires to develop political organizations. The work of these organizers coincided with the help and encouragement Perón gave to the labor unions in his capacity as Secretary of Labor.

9. Perón was arrested (because one military group felt he had become too powerful) in October 1945, and a huge pro-Perón demonstration by workers took place in the historically important central square of the city. This popular manifestation included elements of professional organization, but it also appeared to be at least partly a spontaneous response to the arrest of labor's new hero. The story has been told and retold. One of the original "colonels" (Perón) in the 1943 takeover was carefully organizing labor groups and aiding them in their demands,

which often received legislative backing, but not civil enforcement. This colonel was supporting labor in the name of the government. After the military government arrested Perón, there was a popular (not militarily organized, in a fascist sense—Germani 1962: 248–249) uprising in his support.

10. Perón was released because of his popularity, and several months later he was nominated and elected president of Argentina. The election has been considered one of Argentina's most "honest" elections, and Perón enjoyed the support of both lower- and middle-income groups. Because of popular backing, Perón's rule of Argentina could be described as independent of the military group he had used to launch his political career. Much of his success with the lower-income groups has been attributed to his espousal of existing and new labor legislation and to the popularity of his wife, Evita Duarte de Perón, with the common man.

11. Perón's rule has been called a dictatorship despite the popularity of his candidacy and the great number of votes he received. He nationalized most of the private utilities and pushed reforms designed to help the working class, but he was harsh on intellectuals and organized opposition. Although starting with a fairly prosperous national treasury because of wartime sales of Argentine products, the first administration of Perón began to encounter difficulties in the middle of the term of office. Perón inaugurated a period of militarism and nationalism, including the severe control of academic life and ending with sanctions against the church. By 1951 some military opposition grew but was repressed. Economic difficulties continued. In a military coup of June 1955, Perón was deposed. The constitutional changes instituted by Perón were annulled by a return to the constitution of 1853, and the former president himself was exiled.

12. The provisional government of General Lonardi that began in 1955 was replaced by the provisional presidency of General Pedro Aramburu. In the promised civil elections of 1958, Arturo Frondizi, a member of a Radical party splinter group called the "intransigents," was elected the new president. The Peronist party was declared illegal but was not eliminated, even with it's titular head in exile. Thus Frondizi won many votes by inviting the Peronists to become reincorporated into national political life. Frondizi attempted to reunite the country by appealing to labor with wage boosts and the promise of political representation, to the church by giving Catholic higher education the benefits of the national university system, and to industrialists by obtaining loans permitting imports and allowing foreign investments. In March 1962, after numerous attempted coups, the military removed Frondizi from office (Scobie 1962: 220–221).

13. Although José Guido, was a civilian, the military was considered to dominate the political scene. New elections were called, and in July 1963 Arturo Illia of the conservative wing of the Radical party, became president. Illia's government lasted until June 1966, when General Juan Carlos Onganía, a key military leader at the time of Illia's inauguration in 1963, led a coup and became installed as Argentina's new president. The military continued to rule the country until 1973 when new elections were allowed that swept the peronists back into power. Onganía's coup was accompanied by forceful intervention into the affairs of the university community, and even today the National University of Buenos Aires, one of the best in all Latin America, is a weak institution. Some departments resigned almost outright, and the damage is comparable to that done during the Perón years of government.

14. The Peronists elected Héctor Cámpora as president, but he resigned after a few weeks in office. New elections are scheduled for September 1973 and Perón is expected to be the principal candidate.

The economic picture in Argentina did not improve much after Perón was thrown out. Inflation increased steadily each year, and the gross national product in 1962 was at the same level it had first reached in 1948 (Ferrer 1963: 239). Ferrer estimates that by 1962 the urban masses were approximately 75% of the total Argentine population and that living conditions had not improved between 1948 and 1962, but had actually worsened. Although the Argentines lived rather well in 1948, there was a decline in the standard of living over the next 14 years, which should be emphasized. Ferrer states that by 1962 salaries were 40% lower than they had been in 1948, and various services such as housing, sanitary works, education, and public health had deteriorated. It is this deterioration that the American reader should notice carefully. Americans find it difficult to believe that the United States and Argentina have experienced many parallels in life style, despite the discrepancies that exist in levels of industrialization. Ferrer has remarked that outside observers are often intrigued by Argentina because the country's social and economic structure appears to resemble that of developed countries rather than that of nations which lack development or are stagnated. Ferrer blames much of the arrested growth on the large landowners who, in the 1930s, pushed for a reconstruction of the country's economy along the lines of exporting primary goods rather than by industrialization. He also feels that later political developments led to exaggerated increases in the salaries of the working masses and that the nationalization of foreign-owned corporations was too extensive (1963: 240–241).

According to Ferrer, the government has spent too much time worrying about the more obvious aspects of the economic stagnation (e.g., inflation, deficits) and has not devoted enough attention to the fundamental activities necessary for autonomous growth. Political difficulties continually undercut economic planning and development, leading to contradictory or conflicting policies from one regime to the next. Yet Argentina's standard of living has always been high for a Latin American country. This paradox of maintaining the external appearances of comfort, modernization, and a history of solid cultural and intellectual attainments in the face of continuing economic stagnation gives Argentina the image of a country with unlimited potential yet with a disappointing record of accomplishments when compared with earlier success.

In the view of Germani (1962: 239–252), Argentina grew and moved rapidly from a traditional existence to one in which the condition he labels that of a "mass society" became concretized during Perón's rule. The military takeover of 1930 occurred when the huge external imigration shifted to an internal movement of rural, unskilled workers and their families to the larger cities (1930–1935). These workers were not automatically integrated into the new forms of life they encountered, and there was no meaningful political participation. When the military takeover of 1943 brought Juan Perón onto the scene, the level of internal migration was again beginning to rise, reaching very high proportions between 1950 and 1955. These migrations, which were encouraged by Perón, gave him many potential votes. Perón's organized efforts to attract the masses to his support were made, according to Germani, under totalitarian conditions, thus generating a kind of mass society that endangered the democratic tenets of the constitution. Although certain immediate gains to the worker clearly appeared—such as political participation and social recognition as a valued person—Germani argues that the political organization of workers was superficial and too rapid, while basic civil rights were not available to all. The demagogic appeal of Perón, however, went beyond these newly urbanized masses and included many frustrated middle-class groups whose Radical party leaders had failed to better their situation. The recent military governments have done nothing to break the cycle of sustained inflation and stagnation that has plagued Argentina for more than 40 years.

Several global factors have emerged from the previous discussion to account for Argentina's "greatness" or "success," but never reaching the point of "closure" and never allowing us to say that "success now appears imminent." These global or general "facts" noted earlier include a massive influx of immigrants, with the population increasing 10 times in 90 years—from 1,737,000 in 1869 to an estimated 20,438,000 in 1959 (Germani 1962; 185). This was about double the rate of growth in the United States, Brazil, or Chile, over comparable periods of time. There was an equally rapid shift in the social composition of the population, as fewer people remained dependent on a "boss" or *patron*. Also recorded were huge migrations to the cities, a lowered birth rate, and a shift from a low to a rather high literacy rate. Argentina was one of the few countries of the world in which a major part of its population was foreign-born for several decades (Germani 1965: 209). Despite a long period of enormous economic growth, including advances in sanitary facilities, transportation, and international exchanges, Argentina experienced an economic slowdown between 1920 and 1930, followed by stagnation, which remains today. In addition there was a series of failures to achieve stable, elected representation in government, notwithstanding the introduction of compulsory universal male suffrage in 1912 and suffrage for women in 1947.

The foregoing circumstances suggest to Germani that a politically and socially unintegrated mass of immigrants cannot be absorbed smoothly if the economy does not expand rapidly enough, if the natives do not enjoy political responsibility, and if the population has no confidence in those governing the country. Let me paraphrase Germani's argument. Mass or collective behavior would be likely unless more workers moved from a *patron* relationship with the employer, either rural or urban, to one characterized by more freedom of choice in a larger, more open, labor market, in which demands could be voiced for collective bargaining and employee rights and dignity. Other factors contributing to the "mass society" conditions—increased urbanization and the construction of multiple dwelling units—are accompanied by lower fertility, more women in the labor force, and more education. When we can also note slackened economic development and political instability, and particularly when elected officials are not responsive to public demands, social scientists say that a "mass society," in the popular sense of the term, has been created.

The turning periods in modern Argentine history were (*a*) the period of 1910–1916, when male suffrage was passed, the military was buttressed by the establishment of national conscription (Canton 1965), and the first Radical party candidate for president was elected and (*b*) the period including the second election of Yrigoyen in 1928 and the economic depression that followed, which provided the conservative military coalition with the opportunity to effect a successful coup. This coalition favored previous (oligarchy) policies of political control and economic development; thus it continued to manipulate elections and to stress agricultural expansion and markets at the expense of industrial development. Rather than striving for industrial self-sufficiency, the Argentine economy remained dependent on world food prices.

The military coup of 1930 included high-ranking officers associated with conservatives and low-ranking officers who had their own ideas about the role of the military in Argentine life. The righ-ranking officers came to see themselves as "protectors" of the country against bungling and corrupt civilians.

Coming from mixed socioeconomic origins, the low-ranking officers of the early 1930s became the colonels of the 1940s who took over from the older generals. The colonels orientation toward governing the country did not include realistic economic plans. The group to which Perón belonged seemed to possess a critical awareness of a source of untapped power—the workers and the lower middle classes. The military became established as the bottomless reservoir of leadership in which the only fighting that occurred was between the different branches of service. But there were always civilians who believed that the military's entrance into domestic affairs was justifiable during conditions of domestic unrest. For the military, each civilian government that failed to achieve economic and political stability deserved intervention—an intervention that became more than a military decision insofar as it rested on the notion of civilian dissatisfaction with elected officials.

The emergence of Perón as a strong leader among the colonels, and the apparently careful planning that he devoted to organizing labor to support him, *led to a radical transformation of Argentine society, a a transformation that had been long in the making but which Perón crystallized so dramatically that the initial years of Perón's power in Argentine life could be described as Argentina's only organized "revolution" since colonial days.* The working-class citizen could (and did, much to the disgust of my middle-class informants) walk the streets of Argentine cities feeling that he was an equal to citizens with better paid and "more respected" occupations. One of the leaders of a union local I studied told me that he and other sons of workers could gain entrance to the university during Perón's rule and could easily satisfy the academic requirements for remaining a student. But this man stated that it was very difficult to mix with the overwhelmingly middle- and upper-income students attending the Law School in Buenos Aires. The universities in Argentina remain one stage of a predominantly middle- and upper-income social-ization period preceding adulthood.

No government since 1955 has been able to create a social revolution to parallel the impact of Perón's rule on the political development of the working classes. But increased political consciousness has not prevented continued economic disaster. The Argentine economists have provided considerable information about possible remedies, but two related con-ditions are difficult for Argentines to discuss publicly: (1) the military-conservative coalition and its impact on governmental activities, and (2) the failure of different interest groups (particularly the military) to sacrifice their own social, economic, and political advantages for the good of the country. It is difficult to imagine military groups abolishing their power or abandoning their insistence on the huge budget that maintains a large military complex. Any program of change will create problems, but the military-conservative coalition—a coalition we know little about empirically—is not likely to lead the way with sacrifices.

The series of paradoxes and contrasts that are used to explain Argen-tina's historical development are often difficult for an American to understand. In recent years more Americans have become aware of a number of problems in their own country that could be used as a pro-visional comparative basis for understanding similar problems in Argen-tina. For example, the tremendous cost of American military strength has been linked to United States' involvement in "protective" action all over the world, and the enormous defense budget immediately evokes remarks about the military-industrial complex. The war in Southeast Asia and major defense outlays have seriously affected international stability of the U.S. dollar and have impeded the implementation of urgently needed domestic changes. Like the United States, Argentina con-tinues to spend fortunes for a military network that is difficult to justify when domestic conditions have worsened consistently. Yet in both coun-tries large groups of people defend the military-industrial complex and view it as a "bulwark for freedom." The war in Vietnam and elsewhere in southeast Asia and the racial strife in the United States have intensified among many, feelings of disgust for governmental policies and for the discrepancy that exists between American ideals and practice. This has led some Americans to resist the draft and to emigrate from the country, whereas great numbers have begun to reexamine their patriotism. Simi-larly, Argentines who are dissatisfied with governmental policies and with those who have the power and wealth, make frequent denunciations of their country as the land of the *coima* (bribes). Since Perón's rule, and continuing through recent military governments, emigration has increased, particularly among professional groups. Argentina has been, for some time, an exporter of professionally trained personnel.

The American's image of Argentina (or Latin America) tends to be one of corruption, military dictatorship, and poverty. Yet the American hears daily of corrupt practices in all walks of American life—he hears of political favors, corporate land speculation, price-fixing, and dangerous and fraudulent consumer and health products—which could hardly be described as "minor" in comparison to Latin American activities, for far more money is involved, as well as serious violations of public trust. The poverty of some American inner cities could compete with squalor found in Latin America, although slums in the latter countries often appear to be worse. The feelings of futility with which many Americans confront their loss of faith in government leaders and their handling of military engagements, as well as political corruption and the conditions of poverty and ethnic conflict, have long been standard fare for Argentines. Increasingly, however, strong nationalistic statements are being uttered by the growing numbers of disaffected individuals who remain in Argentina.

Ethnographic Impressions of Buenos Aires.   The number of field and library studies of Latin American countries has increased rapidly during the past 20 years. The studies vary, but most of them report findings obtained from surveys and/or from census or vital statistics materials, as well as from government publications on economic and other activities. The researcher of foreign areas usually relies on a combination of library research and survey work, using local assistants for field contacts with natives, and always devoting at least some time to "living" in the country studied. Research by economists, historians, political scientists, and sociologists seldom includes ethnographic accounts, although some attempt is made to supply a few pages of descriptive remarks about the country's history and current affairs. In writing about a foreign country, most social science specialists restrict their studies to such themes as industrialization, political parties, social stratification, fertility behavior, and gross demographic changes, while avoiding ethnographic description about everyday behavior. Although these studies are not as completely devoid of ethnographic description as are books written about the researcher's own country, the resemblance is unfortunately close. The difficulties of correcting the discrepancies among descriptions about everyday life, abstract theorizing, and so-called hard factual or survey data, are not easily overcome. There is no established precedent, no agreed-upon standard, for describing an entire country or a large urban area—say, Buenos Aires—as a prelude to presenting the presumed "real" data, which may be only a series of tables.

How does one go about writing an ethnography of a city the size of Buenos Aires? I thought about this question during the initial stages of my study, but was soon overwhelmed by the problem and dropped it. Nevertheless, I found myself visiting different parts of the city and its suburbs because of my interviews and those of assistants, and sometimes out of curiosity I examined an area I had been told about. Because I took field notes based on visits to different parts of the city, and because I became involved in two additional smaller studies—socialization practices associated with children who were brought to the municipal children's hospital and diagnosed as psychosomatic, as well as a textile union local—I had written impressions of several types of ecological areas of everyday activity. When I began to draft this book, it became apparent that I was drawing on many of my impressions to elaborate or clarify "findings" that were basic to my original research design. I returned to the problem of How does one write an ethnography of a large city? I feel that the reader will be assisted in interpreting the materials presented if he is exposed to a description of some of my experiences in coming to know the city of Buenos Aires and parts of Argentina. To locate the results of the study within the everyday experiences of the researcher, as well as in a larger historical context, both the history of the country and the contemporary scene seemed to be necessary.

My sample of households was obtained through a variety of sources; chief among them was a probability sample used by Gino Germani for a large study of social stratification in Buenos Aires. Germani's carefully selected sample served as the basic source for my interviews of households, representing large areas of the city and suburban communities. Armed with a map of the city, and accompanied in a chauffer-driven rented car by a research assistant (Ponciano Torales) familiar with the locale, I spent several days exploring the areas from which the households were to be chosen. I took notes as we discussed the areas visited, as we stopped for short walks around a neighborhood, and as we entered various coffee houses for some refreshment and small talk with the bartender and customers. This initial tour proved to be important in exposing me to a huge city. What I saw was rather staggering, however, and I could not absorb nor appreciate the variation until a few months later when I began to revisit the same areas, this time going directly to particular homes where I or my interviewing assistants had already established contact or completed an interview.

My day-to-day contacts with the city were initially restricted to a bus or subway ride downtown and then a few blocks' walk to the University of Buenos Aires, where I was teaching. The buses and subways of Buenos Aires remind me of those in any large city. The atmosphere was impersonal—everyone seemed to be reading a magazine, book, or newspaper—and the density of people was quite noticeable. The majority of buses were fairly small, although great numbers of persons seemed to fit. The buses were called *collectivos* or "collectives" and usually had only one door by the driver. I was struck by the speed at which all buses were driven through the streets and by the passengers' ability to jump off or get on while the bus was still moving. I also noted the number of exchanges, usually unpleasant, between the drivers and the passengers (over the driver's speed, his refusal to stop at a particular street corner, or his refusal to come to a complete stop). The *collectivos* were privately owned and operated on a concession basis, each owner having a particular line or route franchise. The bus was usually brightly painted and the driver's area contained ornaments of a religious nature or perhaps a picture, as a memorial, of Carlos Gardel, the famous Argentine singer of the tango.

STREETS, BUILDINGS, AND SERVICES.   The streets of Buenos Aires reminded me of those in European cities, particularly in Rome and Paris. The architecture had a European cast; and a characteristic feature of buildings was the balcony. All buildings, including apartments and single family units, were flush with the next building, leaving room for windows only in the front and back of the house or apartment. A patio usually provided an open space for apartments that did not front the street. Only corner apartments sometimes afforded windows on two or three sides. Apartment buildings for middle-income people usually housed a *portero* or custodian who maintained the building, received mail, perhaps delivered newspapers, and supplied each family with one or more cases of soda water in siphon bottles. Few buildings of middle-income families contained underground garages, but most had elevators.

Because most buildings fronted flush with the sidewalk and were flush with other buildings on either side, it was not possible to determine what was behind the front door. On opening the front door, for example, one might step into an open area covered by a roof—a kind of porch. Beyond another door might be a patio or the living room. Or, the street door might open onto a long corridor lined with doors on the right side, with a patio attached to the left of the corridor. The doors might lead to separate rooms of one house or to one- or two-room combinations in which entire families lived. The latter arrangement (with many variations) was called a *conventillo,* after the "convent." Some lower- middle-income and many working-class families occupied the *conventillos.* One common pattern was a two- or three-story building that opened from a double door on the street into a short corridor with a few doors leading to rooms. The corridor then opened into a rectangular patio with doors off each side. Each door led to a room occupied by a single family, and there were doors on each level of the building. In another common apartment style, a double or single door on the street opened into a corridor, and there was a narrow patio surrounded by several stories of small apartments. The corridor then continued to another narrow patio and more apartments, perhaps extending 25 to 50 yards or more. The building might extend almost the entire length of the block, but the only part visible from the sidewalk was the façade of the apartments facing the street.

The multiple dwelling units making up most of Buenos Aires are quite crowded because space is at a premium; housing is very difficult to obtain. In *conventillos* two or three generations may never leave their home—one large room, with communal bath and kitchen—located in the heart of downtown Buenos Aires or in a nearby *barrio* or neighborhood. For several decades, migrants from the interior of the country have constructed temporary housing out of sheet metal and wood scraps found in empty lots next to old and new buildings and partially constructed buildings, even in the heart of downtown Buenos Aires. Most of the people in these families have been dark-skinned, dark-haired, poorly educated, and unskilled. The predominantly lighter skinned middle classes call them by the derogatory term *cabecitas negras* or "black heads." In the suburbs (and occasionally in the city, where they were usually walled off) shantytown slums (*villas miserias*) were commonly encountered. Families have settled in open fields, around refuse dumps, or inside and outside abandoned factories or public buildings. Many of these residences have electricity (stolen from public or private lines), and there are even a few telephones—the instrument having been purchased by mail order and shared with relatives, friends, or neighbors.

A striking feature of all buildings in Buenos Aires is their poor state of repair. It is difficult to provide good maintenance because of inflationary costs and because construction supplies and fixtures frequently must be imported. Many public buildings are carefuly cleaned inside, but the constant use of water and strong cleansing agents has only served to accelerate the deterioration of old parts, fixtures, tiles, and wooden floors. This effect is visible in all municipal hospitals. Whereas the medical services are usually quite good thanks to well-trained physicians, the buildings, equipment, and medical supplies are in poor repair or not available. The federal customs service is so badly corrupted by bribery (*coima*), that even municipal hospitals have difficulties importing badly needed medical equipment and supplies. My primary (though not only) experience with hospitals was in the large municipal Hospital de Niños (Children's Hospital), where I obtained a number of interviews with people from the *villas miserias*. The medical treatment seemed to vary in sophistication from ward to ward, but many wards provided highly competent physicians, for minimal or no cost, in rather drab, depressing surroundings. The picture I developed seemed to be familiar in Argentina, and particularly in Buenos Aires; the high standards and often the extravagances of some 30 to 50 years ago have not been maintained, and the Argentine's dream of the good life is continually spoiled by the worsening appearances all around him, which serve as reminders of past achievements and present realities.

From about 1910 to 1930, Buenos Aires could be compared quite favorably with New York, London, Stockholm, Berlin, Paris, and Rome, as the public works (sanitation, water purification, broad streets, parks, etc.) , the public transportation system (subways, commuter trains) , and cultural and educational attainments reached high levels and justified national pride. The level of "modernity" remains high enough today to warrant describing Buenos Aires as one of the world's great cities, but the deterioration and stagnation and the reminders of past achievements intensifies the cynicism of the *porteño's* (dweller of Buenos Aires) everyday conversation.

Even the streets and sidewalks convey the "broken dream" atmosphere —utility or sewer repairs are made, but the finishing touches, such as the replacement of ceramic tiles, asphalt, or cobblestones, are always uneven in degree of completion or quality of material. In addition to coping with the dense human and automotive traffic in many sections of the city, the pedestrian in Buenos Aires may have to maneuver around rubble, manholes, and detour signs.

Although many streets of Buenos Aires were laid out with regard for use of space and landscaping, the same amount of planning and care has not been sustained over the years. Nor have the public services kept pace—all reflect the deterioration problem, against a backdrop of *prior* elegance or quality. Telephones are difficult to obtain (except after long waits or bribes) and do not always function adequately. Electricity has long been a basic service, and at one time was on a par with North American and European standards, but the demand has increased far beyond the utility's ability to expand. Every winter frequent breakdowns have left some districts without lights, elevators, and other services for hours. The railroads have been a national economic disaster for years, and the quality of railroad equipment and services varies considerably.

The most noteworthy feature of public services and public bureaucracies in Argentina (and throughout Latin America and southern Europe) is that there are more employees than are required to perform the actual work (a kind of featherbedding). This padding of the labor force in public bureaucracies, including the military, helps to keep unemployment rates lower, particularly over periods of long economic stagnation, but it also increases the number of persons who are eligible for public pensions. According to many informants, the excess of workers leads to shorter working hours, less output, and less pay because of inflation and because of obstacles to higher wages. The serious consequence is that many must seek a second and even a third job to maintain their families. Public service employees told me that they tried to work less on their main job to conserve their energy for their second and/or third position.

Informants were quick to note that is is rather difficult to dismiss a public employee. Paradoxically, Argentina has always sustained large public bureaucracies despite an absence of the kind of industrialization usually associated with service industries in developed countries. The large service-oriented labor force is the sign of a costly and inefficient bureaucracy, rather than an index of economic development. Such a situation could be described as urbanization that does not reflect economic development, although it still contains elements of "modernization."

In summary, Argentina is a country that has long been modern and urbanized, but economically and politically stagnant—the statement is especially true of its capital, Buenos Aires. Cultural activities flourish, and Argentina continutes to be a major exporter of professional expertise (physicians, dentists, engineers, physicists, musicians, artists, writers, etc.). Much of the indifference and cynicism of the *porteño* is probably a reflection of the "big city" complex researchers tend to use when describing our impressions of urban living. But in Buenos Aires, as in New York City, considerable bitterness seemed to accompany remarks that are roughly equivalent to the North American expression, "You can't fight City Hall."

EDUCATION.   I first visited elementary schools on behalf of my preschool children and my school age child. In later months I looked for a local state school for the eldest. I visited several private schools and a few neighborhood state schools. The more expensive private schools had more attractive physical plants and newer buses. The instruction in the private schools was usually bilingual (e.g., Spanish-English, Spanish-Italian, etc.). Special uniforms were mandatory, and a blazer jacket was the distinctive feature. The students were picked up in the morning by bus, some as early as 7:00 or 7:30 A.M., and returned between 4:30 and 6:00 P.M. Each student, including those in kindergarten, carried a briefcase filled with papers, books, pencils, toys, and snacks for recess periods. The school schedule was often long and difficult for the children. I gathered that the school served some parents as a convenient baby sittter and as a socializing force. With the father returning from work between 8:00 and 9:00 P.M., the child's primary contacts outside school were with the maid or servant (*mucama*) and the mother. Some middle-income families sent their children to a state school until noon, when the session ended, and then to a private school for second language instruction in the afternoon.

I visited about five state schools; all were in need of repairs, were rather old, and usually lacked teaching materials. The teachers, who were not well paid, complained about poor heating in the rooms and about the lack of teaching aids and supplies. All the students wore white shirts and neckties, as in the private schools, and white smocks over their clothes. In both the state and private schools it was customary for the teachers to assign homework virtually every day, even in the first grade. The state school students also carried their briefcases, which seemed very heavy to me.

I was not overly impressed with state elementary education in Buenos Aires, although it certainly seemed to be equivalent to state elementary education in the United States. The Argentine high schools—particularly a few in Buenos Aires, and especially the National High School, which is connected to the state university—seemed to be better than North American high schools, however. The level of instruction in physical and biological sciences and in literature seemed to be more advanced, and the students were more self-reliant. As the reader will realize, I have no convincing evidence of the difference in quality, but I feel that it is important to indicate the impression I formed. I knew a number of high school students, and I used to ask them about their work in courses. I occasionally examined their textbooks, and I spoke to a few instructors about the level of the instructors' education.

To me the most remarkable difference between public schools in Argentina and in the United States is in the physical plants. The North Americans place considerable emphasis on appearances, whereas Argentina's economic stagnation seems to prevent a similar concern. Yet I do not feel that the quality of instruction in Argentina suffers because of the poor plant facilities.

Earlier I indicated that the student body in Argentine universities seemed to come primarily from middle-income families. Most courses were given in the late afternoon and evening, and dress was rather formal, as it was in all public activities. There was far less emphasis than in American universities on completing a program of courses leading to the degree within a fixed time—say, four years. However, students were quite segregated by their particular field of interest and had less contact with students in other disciplines than American students do. The physical conditions reflected impoverishment; classroom facilities were minimal and in poor repair, and libraries fell considerably below the lowest American standards. Library resources might be enhanced during the tenure of a particular dean or department chairman, but there were few books and no study space under the best of circumstances. Many professors and serious students had to develop their own libraries, for there was no central university library, nor even a municipal or national library, where the student might find books relevant to his studies. Final examinations, administered by the professor and two outside instructors, were usually individual and given orally, but the entire class could witness the performance. The student's final grade was negotiated and decided at the end of the examination, with the professor entering the grade on a card that went to the administration and on the student's personal record, which was returned to him immediately.

During my stay in Buenos Aires the university scene became more and more politicized within departments, and internal political divisions influenced general policy decisions and administrative activities in which students and faculty members had a voice. My impressions led me to conclude that because of political activities, many of the students were not interested in serious studying, yet they did seem to want to be able to say that they had a university degree or title. Thus many students alleged that some courses were "too difficult," and some highly active student leaders apparently took advantage of this complaint by stirring up students against professors and their courses. Organized efforts were made to discredit professors and courses, and attempts were made to influence the choice in hiring of assistants and faculty. This situation intensified after I left Buenos Aires on July 1, 1964, and during subsequent visits in 1968, 1969, and 1972, I noted that the trend was becoming even stronger. The new military government that began in June 1966 used the "extremist" influence and disruption as its justification for intervention in all university affairs. But the intervention also led to questioning the authority of a very large group of serious professors and assistants, if not discrediting them altogether. Thus the military government could rid itself of most of the troublemakers—which meant the extremists, in their conservative view—even though the group labeled "troublemakers" had been conveniently expanded to include nonextremist assistants and professors. Many of the nonextremist personnel, who had originally given the university its academic prominence, now resigned. Activist students were interested in their ideological goals, not in fighting the government for more budgetary allowances, more pay for assistants and professors, better teaching facilities, and higher quality instruction. The mass of students seemed to be manipulated by small groups of highly active leaders who used the university to attack national policies and inequities as well as university activities. The extremist group opposed the attempts made by some students, younger assistants, and professors to improve the curriculum and the quality of instruction. Many student leaders of all political persuasions were older than the average undergraduate; these individuals prolonged their education for years, maintaining student status by registering for a minimal number of courses. In attacking policies and persons, extremist students often painted slogans on walls or hung open letters and posters inside and outside the buildings. Frequently seniority of service as a student teaching assistant, research assistant, or junior faculty member was more important in career improvement (as reflected in pay demands made) than such criteria as teaching ability, higher degrees, advanced study, and research experience and publications.

Students in all fields had to contend with a tight labor market after graduation, but most of those in the humanities and social sciences had to look for work in other fields.

There were many political divisions within the faculty and among students, and as a rule the divisions were public. A person's academic interests were usually tied to political associations that had begun during formative years in high school and college. In Buenos Aires a first year undergraduate student (who begins to specialize immediately in his chosen major—e.g., physics, sociology, biology, psychology) is drawn into some part of the existing political divisions, and this initial commitment may become the basis for long-term political allegiances. Thus a visiting professor or student who develops friendships with the one group may find that others are no longer friendly to him and that discussions of academic matters are influenced accordingly. Academic interests also structure the visitor's (and the native's) social and political encounters. If the visitor tries to straddle two or more groups, he may find that he has few friends and little or no social exchanges with natives, or that the exchanges he does have remain superficial.

EVERYDAY INTERACTION.   At the time of my study, Argentines employed a European pattern of acquaintance formation. Use of first names was rather restricted and often limited to persons who were peers and had become friends before their occupational careers had commenced. Various uses of formal greetings and identifications seemed to serve as possible barriers to intimacy. The use of titles was customary (though not as in Mexico, where anyone who has graduated from a university is addressed both orally and in writing as *licenciado*), particularly among engineers, architects, physicians, and dentists. Often a title or Señor, Señorita, or Senora was all that was used, or the title and the last name. There was also frequent use of the last name only. Thus an oral greeting would be "Hola López," and during the conversation the usage would be "But look López, you can't. . . ." Letters begin with "Estimado López," a practice found in Europe and in the United States, some 30 or 40 years ago.

For Argentines the "intimate" use of last names might still be accompanied by formal address forms and third person verb conjugations. For Americans there seemed to be a paradox involved in learning to like someone; the American might invite someone to his house, be invited to that individual's house in return, and feel that he and the other person liked each other. The American and his Latin American friends might greet one another with a warm embrace, or with simulated kisses in the case of females, yet many Latin friends still call the American "Dear Jones." The conversations I found most paradoxical were multiparty conversations, or those in which a cordial last-name usage was established and the discussion included references to a person known to one or both parties on a first name (called *tutear*) basis. Here it was necessary to use the last name with one party and the first name with a second party; alternatively, I myself was either the "last name" or "first name" party, depending on the speaker. In both situations a sharp shift from familiar to polite grammatical verb forms (or vice versa) was necessary. It was the familiarity or distance attached to the use of verb forms that made the conversation seem confusing.

Some informants indicated that one or two generations ago children always addressed their parents with the third person singular and plural verb and subject forms, but this has been changing. Married couples always seemed to use the familiar form of address. In American English it is possible to avoid grammatical reminders of formality and social distance, but the reminders are built into the Spanish language. In American English it is common to use polite forms of address, but the Spanish introduces important social distinctions because the sharp distinction between polite and familiar is built into all communication so that formality is revealed through the use of pronouns and verb conjugation. It is only when a title and/or last name is used that the American feels the formality. The use of pronouns and verb conjugations in American English does not remind the speaker-hearer of the formality that may or may not exist. In Spanish the pronouns and verbs remain in polite form and serve as markers to the participants, continually emphasizing the social distance between them. I found that the pronouns and verb forms were constant reminders because I had to make an effort to remember to produce comparable polite forms. This made me a little tense at times because the polite forms obscured my normal ways of deciding that someone was "friendly," "cold," "interested," and the like. I found myself hesitating to use certain expressions for fear of offending the other party.

My feeling is that language problems of this type punctuate all comparative research, but researchers seldom know how to reveal the impact of language on research procedures and on the analysis of findings. The researcher finds it difficult to evaluate his participation in daily encounters with natives. Hence the feedback he receives from the communication does not permit him to judge how his questions are interpreted by the subject. It is not clear to the researcher whether the questions asked and the responses given are free from distortions and ambiguities, which a native might compensate for adequately when speaking to another native. The researcher's ability to adjust to communication problems improves with time, but it is impossible to estimate how much he has lost in terms of meaning throughout different stages of an interview or during the entire research period. I found that during subsequent research in Mexico I had become more able to use polite forms freely, and I attributed much of my "improvement" to my lectures at the University of Buenos Aires, which required the relentless use of the polite forms of Spanish. When I made mistakes in the use of language forms, I was reminded to sharpen my speech, and I acquired some impressions about the effects of misuse. If I misspoke to a native, for example, I detected a brief shift in the eyes and a slight pause in the response, as if the other party were trying to assess the significance of my error. I decided that such changes in the native speaker's attitude could mean that I was being viewed as "rude," "ignorant," or "intimate." Such reactions served to make me very self-conscious about my speech and at times tense and uncomfortable.

Another complication of everyday interaction during field work has to do with the physical distance used in conversation. Argentines stand closer to each other while talking than do Americans. This close proximity to the speaker seemed necessary to Argentines and other Latins, but was confusing to me: I was obliged to be very self-conscious about using polite forms of address at the same time that I was standing in a close, and to me familiar, way. Close physical proximity of the speakers does not seem to be part of the structure of routine exchanges in the United States. The subtleties of face-to-face communication in various countries have not been described empirically on a comparative basis, and one does not become clearly aware of the tacit rules employed in the familiar everyday scenes of his own community, much less in a foreign country.

The formalities I have touched on occurred in interactions among middle-income persons and between persons from middle-income families and persons from lower-income families. Among the unskilled, semi-skilled, and skilled workers of a textile union which I observed for some five months, the use of the familiar seemed to be routine, and newly introduced workers often asked for the first name of the other person if a conversation proved lengthy and friendly. I noticed, however, that it was very difficult for me to go beyond a "friendly" last-name basis with the union leaders and workers who spent leisure time in the union's bargaining office area of the factory or in the union's own offices a few blocks away. During heated discussions people occasionally switched from the polite to the familiar when addressing me. This usually occurred when a person had been directing his remarks to a fellow worker and then had shifted his conversation to me. If the worker discovered the switch he often appeared embarrassed. I was the only one present with whom the polite form was used, however, and it was difficult for many of the workers to use both forms when conversing in a group (Gumperz and Blom: 1971).

FAMILY LIFE.   My impressions of Argentine family life in Buenos Aires were obtained during frequent visits to homes where I interviewed one or both parents, or during my visits to a home where a research assistant had completed an interview or had encountered difficulties.

Working-class homes were usually cramped for space. The father was seldom there; he was either working or passing his time at the neighborhood bar, which might serve coffee, tea, soft drinks, beer, wine, or liquor. The men sitting in bars devoted most of their conversation to sports and women. One of the few telephones in the neighborhood was usually located in the bar. Occasionally the bar was used by a couple as a meeting place, and many bars (though more in business districts than in neighborhoods) had a special section for families or couples. In some bars the special section was distinguished by tablecloths and perhaps nicer furniture.

Middle-income bars or barlike establishments were more often patronized by couples who appeared to be unmarried persons with no other place to meet. I gathered that the male in Argentina, particularly the middle-income male, did not have to account for his time to his wife (as contrasted with the middle-income male in the United States). Since only relatives and close friends were entertained at home, married couples often went out for the evening when entertaining guests, and parties or wedding celebrations were frequently held in a hotel or restaurant.

The lower-income wife spent most of the day cleaning the house, making numerous trips to the neighborhood stores for small purchases. Upper-middle-income and some middle-income wives directed their servants in cleaning the house and sent a servant on many minor errands. They went to the beauty parlor often, met friends for lunch, visited relatives, and the like.

The middle class in Argentina (including several provinces I visited) seemed to me to differ from comparable segments of the American population. I have already mentioned the independence of the Argentine husband and his minimal contact with his children. The availability of live-in servants at low cost was probably mainly responsible for the first feature. All middle-income housing seemed to have servants' quarters, and most of the apartment houses I visited had separate entrances for the servants. The use of servants allowed both husband and wife more time away from home and meant less mutual monitoring of their respective activities. Families often went on vacation accompanied by one or more servants.

LABOR. Throughout my stay in Argentina the newspapers published commentaries by military authorities about the dangers of the *Peronistas* (followers of Perón). Yet the newspapers also reported that the labor unions (presumedly composed of followers of Perón) were badly divided. Hence they were hardly a unified force, following the orders of the (then) exiled Perón.

My association with workers and labor unions was primarily based on research in a textile union local. The following remarks outline some general facts and a few of my experiences. In May 1964 the C.G.T. (Argentina's General Confederation of Labor) launched a previously announced plan to obtain higher wages and other benefits. According to newspaper accounts, this *plan de lucha or* "battle plan" was led by the "peronist dominated directorate of the C.G.T." The strategy was to pressure management to yield to demands for higher wages and fringe benefits by staging a series of worker takeovers of various factories for increasingly longer periods of time, but only in terms of hours. The workers allegedly took "hostages," but there were no serious incidents or violence. Prior to the so-called battle plan, a general protest march and assembly was organized in front of the national congress in the Congressional Square, a rather large area in a busy section of Buenos Aires. Estimates of the size of the crowd varied, but some claimed 50,000 participants. The leaders of the C.G.T. had come to protest officially about the worker's conditions and to present their demands.

The workers belonging to textile unions were to proceed by bus from factories, assembling in front of the union headquarters, which was located near the square where the protest was to be held. From there they would march together to the rally. The day before the march, when I asked the local president of the textile union local how many buses had been ordered to take workers to the headquarters, I was told that only four buses would be ordered because a poor turnout was expected. In fact, the local president stated it would take some effort to fill the buses with 200 workers.

The next day, as 5000 workers poured out of the factory early as part of the work stoppage connected with the march, the local president, the secretary, the treasurer, and the elected delegates governing the union local, all began to grab workers they knew to urge them into the buses parked across the street. With some effort they filled the buses. Huge signs praising the "battle plan" were mounted on the sides of the buses. I joined the local president on one of the buses and we proceeded to the headquarters of the union. We parked a few blocks away, and the signs from the bus were attached to long poles. After assembling, we marched as a group to the headquarters. There was a very large crowd in front of the building housing the executive offices of the union. The head of the union, Framini, appeared at a window. He was dressed casually in a brown sport shirt and slacks, and the crowd provided a few mild cheers.

We all marched down the street in the direction of the Congressional Square, turned up one block, and entered the normally very busy street Entre Rios (now empty of cars, although some curious onlookers lined the sidewalks). As we marched down the street singing songs about Perón, apartment windows were closed, businesses locked their doors, and iron shutters were dropped. The square was heavily congested, and we moved to a location away from the congressional building but remained together. Throughout the program, which was directed by union leaders from the congressional building, we stood around, drank coffee purchased from mobile vendors, and spoke about politics, sports, and women. It was difficult to hear the speakers, and although singing occasionally broke out, there was no violence—aside from a few noise bombs that exploded in the nearby subway. The leaders of the march told all the women and the *norteamericano* to stay in the center as we moved out toward the location of our buses. Everyone seemed to be concerned about moving safely away from the scene.

Throughout the demonstration the leaders of various locals met together to complain about the difficulties of convincing more workers to join the march. I was impressed with the extensive apathy among the Peronists both at the rank and file level and among the various leaders I met. Many complaints were directed at the top union leaders, who were described as "corrupt" and only interested in personal power, rather than in the plight of the worker. Yet, as some local leaders noted, the top leaders at least *sounded* "militant" and perhaps could "scare" the government; that is, it was perceived that threatening was better than doing nothing. The papers reported friction between Peronist dominated workers (who were in the majority and were presumably split by Augusto Vandor of the metallurgical union, and Andrés Framini of the textile union), and a smaller group of unions called the "independents."

On the next day several newspapers published denunciations of the protest by a high-ranking general, who claimed that the march had been a dangerous indication of Peronist power and evil intentions. The newspapers described the demonstration as an example of Peronist power and disregard for "law and order." Many military leaders had criticized the government's ineptness in allowing "unlawful" demonstrations by labor groups or had claimed that the government was not forceful enough in blocking demonstrations or in controlling them once in progress. Thus the military, according to newspaper accounts, accused the government of being "weak" because it allowed the Peronists to organize "incidents"; hence the government was incapable of controlling the events it allowed to happen. And the military could provide its own justification for, at some point, entering the scene with another coup. This kind of talk was common in the mass media and in everyday conversations throughout my stay in Argentina. In speaking with students and faculty at the university, with physicians at the Children's Hospital, and with neighbors and respondents from my fertility study, I was impressed with the degree of power attributed to the Peronist group. There was a continual reference to a "they," as if everyone were talking about a coherent, integrated, organized force.

My impression that the unions were apathetic and divisive, despite public imputations of "power," was reinforced a few weeks later when the battle plan began to include additional work stoppages. The leaders of the textile local I was observing objected to having their factory included because the pay scale, already high, was about to be restudied jointly by management and labor, and work conditions were rather favorable. There were heated exchanges between the leaders of the local and the officers of the parent textile organization. The local agreed to have its factory included, but the president of the local told me that he met with the management and worked out a cooperative "takeover," including white-collar "hostages" who would continue to work. My observations of the demonstration at the factory led me to conclude that a kind of carnival atmosphere existed, despite the presence of the police under riot-readiness conditions and despite huge signs proclaiming the "takeover" by the union. Women workers were flirting with police officers and throwing coins down to the street to enable the police to buy them snacks from mobile vendors. There were no incidents, and a "successful" operation was proclaimed. The next day the newspapers were again talking about the danger inherent in the situation and the possibility that the occupations could end in a "revolution." The newspapers' references to the dangerous climate that existed and to the alleged power of the unions (which in fact were without strike funds and were quite divided) were often accompanied by vague comments by a general that the armed forces might intervene. While the unions threatened the government, the military threatened both—and held all the organized power.

The textile union was split by many internal conflicts, including allegations reported to me by members of union locals that the top leaders were squandering funds, that doctors and nurses at the clinic located in the union headquarters building were not receiving their paychecks, and that local leaders were not adequately consulted about general policy issues. The local I studied had hired its own doctor and dentist and housed them in its local office, to provide its workers with better treatment and to ensure the payment of the professionals. This indicates that conditions in individual factories and local unions were usually quite varied, such that isolated cases of better labor–management relations were another source of strain with the national textile union.

I was able to observe union problems in another context during two long bargaining sessions over a new contract between textile union officials and management representatives. I was allowed to attend the meetings as if I were a union member. I was impressed with the discrepancy in the appearances of the two groups. The workers' group consisted of a few full-time officials and a larger number of local representatives who had been given time off from work to attend the meeting. These workers were dressed in a variety of clothing styles—there was a mixture of old suits with dark sport shirts, sport shorts and sweaters with work trousers, or sport shirts, neckties, work trousers, and an old coat that remained from a previous suit. The union officials in the workers' group, who were somewhat better dressed, wore old suits, old-looking business shirts, and neckties. In comparison, the management officials were turned out like stereotypes of the Wall Street banker.

The two groups sat on opposite sides of a long table, and a government moderator sat at the head of the table. The moderator was weak and ineffective; both management and labor officials ignored him when angry and simply interrupted whoever was speaking, not waiting for recognition by the moderator. The management representatives said very little during the exchanges; they spoke softly and would not budge from their position. The union representatives were very talkative, very loud, and emotional. During the second meeting negotiations broke down when the leader of the union group launched a heated attack on the management group, which he characterized as "flunkies" who could not really speak for their superiors, claiming that they had not come to bargain but merely to provide token evidence of negotiation while holding to a rigid

and unfair management line on wages, fringe benefits, and work conditions. The union official was an emotional but eloquent speaker and had
been close to Perón during and after the latter's rule. The management
group walked out after this verbal onslaught.

I was told by two informants from the union group that their particular locals (including the one I had studied) were not always in agreement with the Peronist union official's position because their dealings
with management had been friendly and profitable. But the two informants supported the leader at the meeting because of union loyalty and
because of the poor conditions of the majority of workers at most of the
other factories. Both local union and management officials of the factory
I studied maintained their respective loyalties at the meeting while
tacitly recognizing their cooperation outside of the meetings.

My union informants insisted that the labor groups were all divided
because of local and national differences in leadership views, power, and
ambitions. I gathered that most of the union's activities were undermined
because of internal conflicts, a lack of financial support for work stoppages, and general corruption. The union's threat was chiefly a bluff
that was perpetuated by all to allow for some leverage with the public
and military–governmental circles. My informants insisted that the
union's activities were not politically relevant for gaining power to
influence governmental operations and that their only hope was grass
roots political participation in the respective communities with the party
identified as Peronist. The political organizations of their *barrios* and
worker suburbs were active despite continual obstacles to legitimacy and
participation posed by military-dominated governments. Union activities
were considered to be ritualistic performances engaged in for the sake
of appearances.

COMPARATIVE RESEARCH PROBLEMS. I have presented some historical
notes and general impressions of Buenos Aires to delimit my knowledge
and to furnish some background materials that will aid the reader in
locating data appearing in subsequent chapters. I have tried to select a
few areas I felt were critical to an understanding of the contemporary
scene. I did not discuss, for example, the military or religious milieus
because I had virtually no contact with military or church officials.

As soon as a researcher enters an area in which he is obviously a
foreigner, his ignorance about everyday life becomes very apparent.
Leaving the path of the tourist makes one more aware of his foreignness
because of reactions from natives when he asks for directions in local

neighborhoods and enters bars and restaurants which tourists seldom frequent. If the researcher is initially taken to be a native, the conversation may be incomprehensible, because of slang usage, rapid speech, and the truncated syntactic constructions used by the native. When the native decides that he is speaking to a foreigner, however, he begins to alter his presentation by, for example, speaking more slowly and using more complete grammatical constructions and less or no slang.

Being recognized and treated as a foreigner in local neighborhoods requires sensitive communications that a tourist may never need to cope with. If one is not recognized as a foreigner and routine talk occurs, he may appear to be a rather stupid native. This sometimes happened to me late in my stay, when I had adopted a fairly convincing *porteño* accent but missed some slang expressions and hence the gist of certain brief dialogues.

Assuming that anthropological studies have emphasized this point on many occasions, I have said nothing about the advantages of being a foreigner. I am more concerned with the disadvantages due to the tendency in field research to be misled by one's increasing interest in learning how to see things as a native sees them. The advantages of the stranger are many, particularly when a study is first started. My impression is that the advantages of being a stranger may be short-lived if the researcher attempts to immerse himself too quickly in his daily round of activities.

I would like to underscore the following points.

1. Even with a good working knowledge of the language, the researcher, literally does not "see" and "hear" as the native does; therefore, he is continually receiving selective inputs and truncated bits of information, leading to partial understanding of an action scene.

2. As the researcher struggles to set up his research project he must make important judgments about the native culture—judgments that influence his gathering of data and the kind of tacit knowledge he can bring to bear on the analysis of the data. Throughout the research experience, judgments about what a neighborhood is like, about the sincerity of a respondent, or about the adequacy of an answer, are dependent on the researcher's changing conception of the native culture.

3. When speaking to foreign researchers, natives will alter their remarks to allow for presumed gaps in the researcher's knowledge or for his ignorance. Although this accommodation may mean that the native takes more pains to get a point across, it also means the native will decide that some things are not worth saying because they are "too complicated."

4. As the researcher improves his language ability and his knowledge

of everyday practices (both for simple survival and as data), the research materials gathered are being defined according to his state of knowledge or ignorance at such different stages. Thus large amounts of structured information are obtained at particular stages of field research, and as the character of the researcher's experiences changes over time, new meanings are added because of his changing background. Later on, perhaps months or years later, when "the data"—now treated as atemporally relevant—are analyzed and assembled into tables and descriptive propositions, the researcher's findings almost always ignore the fact that he has acquired "the data" from a perspective that has been altered by structured and time-bound field notes and by his memory of "what it was like." "What it was like" is now attributed to the structured and time-bound data as if the present memory of experiences is adequate for elaborating the truncated materials called data. The interpretation of the time-bound data is done in a *here and now* that is a historicized version of what was experienced when the "facts" were recorded.

5. The researcher can seldom master the area's language to the level of native competency. Thus he can seldom perceive the information available from native respondents at a level deeper than the surface sense, much less communicate his intentions to the native when some departure from a literally translated questionnaire is required.

6. The researcher cannot present the "findings," whether "hard" or "soft," in a sterile, atemporal, context-free vacuum under the assumption that he is being rigorous or "scientific." The presentation of findings must reveal the historical context and the temporally induced transformations that have influenced the interpretation of data.

CHAPTER 4

Some General Characteristics of the Study

This chapter is a broad presentation of my impressions of the life styles of the households visited, as well as an introduction to a few characteristics of the survey. I briefly indicate how the results of the survey can lead to different interpretations of fertility behavior and family organization.

General Impressions. The sample actually interviewed (Table 1) was selected by using Gino Germani's larger probability sample (Table 2). Germani had divided the Greater Buenos Aires area into zones, selecting a predetermined quota at random. Germani kindly provided the information in Table 2 and access to the house listings by street and number (or comparable identification when no number existed) and zone. I did not choose the same households sampled by Germani, of course, but contiguous or nearby blocks were selected. At least two or more houses were selected in each zone, depending on the density of the population in the area. I did not attempt to make this a precise process but used it merely as a guide for ensuring that a few cases from most of the zones were included in the final sample. The final selection of zones was based on the advice of different Argentine graduate assistants familiar with the city and on my own observations obtained from riding around the city and familiarizing myself with the type of home and the general appearance of different neighborhoods. I took notes as we drove around the city and relied on comments from one assistant and occasionally on the knowledge of the driver of our rented car. In addition, we stopped for coffee and to query local residents on certain gross characteristics of the

TABLE 1.   SOCIOECONOMIC STATUS OF THE FAMILIES INTERVIEWED[a]

Socioeconomic Status Level[b]	Frequency	Percentage
1	6	3.5
2	48	28.2
3	49	28.7
4	32	18.7
5	18	10.5
6	15	8.8
7	3	1.7
Total	171	100.1

[a] 252 cases in main sample.
[b] In this tabulation, 1 represents the lowest socioeconomic status; 7, the highest.

TABLE 2.   SOCIOECONOMIC STATUS OF GERMANI'S RESPONDENTS

Socioeconomic Status Level[a]	Frequency	Percentage
1	87	4.2
2	778	37.5
3	583	28.1
4	379	18.3
5	159	7.7
6–7	87	4.2
Total	2073	100.0

[a] In this tabulation, 1 represents the lowest socioeconomic status; 6–7, the highest.

neighborhoods (e.g., transportation, shopping, and general occupational activities of residents).

An examination of Table 1 reveals that the lower- and middle-income groups were strongly represented in our sample, whereas the lowest (*villa miseria* or shantytown families) and the highest groups were not heavily represented. Table 2 indicates a fairly similar pattern for Germani's sample, although there is a higher representation of working-class households. My work was limited in scope, but it constituted a detailed study of a small number of families believed to be characteristic of the Argentine scene.

Argentina has been described as having a large middle-income group, as well as a working-class group whose standard of living overlaps that of the lower middle-income group. But these distinctions of social class can provide the reader only with rough ideas about Argentina. Encoded measurements of social class are implicit indicators because the behavioral activities of each class grouping remain gross depictions. The constructed statistical-type measures have been seldom articulated clearly with ethnographic descriptions of day-to-day behavior. The tables on social class were assembled, therefore, as a shorthand way of convincing the reader that the sample being used to present descriptions of fertility and family organization in Argentina is "representative." "Representative" means, however, that quasi-arbitrary measures of occupation, income, education, housing facilities, and material possessions, were forced into a traditional sociological index. Measures of social class have been used as convenient sociological constructions designed to meet abstract structural notions of social stratification, but they are not wholly satisfactory.

For example, descriptions of Argentine social class based on general appearances would not reveal that many families remained in old neighborhoods where rents were low, preferring to spend the money saved on consumer luxuries or on vacations. Many families in high rent neighborhoods lived in old buildings that the owners would not repair because of rent control; yet the tenants would not fix up the premises because of possible changes in rent control laws. Some further general description might clarify my impressions of different life styles.

The lowest income group included persons living in *villas miserias,* in which a labyrinth of dirt paths runs within a variable area of one or more city blocks. The paths occasionally crisscrossed the interior of the area and were often littered with garbage, papers, bottles, and tin cans. The *villas miserias* primarily contained shacks, although there were a few permanent constructions around the periphery. The shacks usually housed one family apiece, and there was sometimes a communal toilet (a jerry-built outhouse) for a group of shacks. One group of shacks might be separated from another by a fence, and each was reached by a path and had a different entrance to the area. The floors of the shacks were dirt, wood, or cement.

The interiors may be heated by a small, upright gas stove fueled by a portable tank of gas. One seldom finds more than one or two small windows (and these usually in the "better" *villas*). Furniture might include a table and a couple of chairs, a radio, and even a television set.

Electricity could be "borrowed" by illegally hooking up with other lines. Running water was usually available at a common tap outside the villa, on a street corner, or in a nearby block. The inhabitants' clothes, however, were usually indistinguishable from those of lower-middle-income or traditional working-class families.

Many of the families were from Paraguay, Bolivia, or Chile, bringing elements of rural living from these countries. Thus I noted that their life style was often similar to that of Argentine families from the north. The children always seemed to be suffering from head and chest colds. The women usually worked as maids and the men as day laborers. Common-law marriages seemed to be routine, with many of the woman's or man's kin visiting on weekends or in the evenings at mealtime. Informants reported that a man often objected to the wife's relatives coming around to "steal" meals when he was working. Since the man's attachment to the woman and children could be weak and temporary, the children could call different men "father" over a period of a few years. These common-law marriage arrangements produced difficult kinship relations—the children only met their maternal kin because the father was not willing to expose the children to his relatives. The wife's problem was to hold on to the "husband" long enough for him to contribute to the support of the household while the children were growing up. "Holding on" could entail providing the man with sexual satisfaction on demand, a bed, food, and clean clothes in good repair, as well as relieving him of most if not all responsibility in raising the children. The father did not participate in the few family outings that occurred, but the activity was likely to include maternal kin. Occasional visits during vacation periods and holidays, therefore, were maternally oriented.

A second qualitative level or style of life in Buenos Aires at the time of our study could be termed *conventillo* living, where existing older buildings or single dwelling units were subdivided into overcrowded living accommodations. There were a wide variety of *conventillos*, but most of my experience was limited to one common type, which formerly had been a single dwelling unit. As mentioned previously, the front door of the original house opened directly onto the sidewalk. On entering, one walked into an open patio with separate, but sometimes connecting, rooms strung along one or both sides of the patio. Another type was a large, several-story apartment building, constructed around a central patio. It was common to find one family per room in *conventillos*, although occasionally a family acquired an adjacent room or a second room in aonther part of the building. As in the case of *villas miserias,* there

was constant contact between neighbors, and because a restricted terri-
torial area was shared and guarded jointly, neighbors often developed
considerable mutual trust. In any event, relatives or friends, invited or
uninvited, lived in the same area. Security did not seem to be a serious
problem inside the housing area because it was very rare for all the
members of a family to be gone at the same time.

General hygiene standards (in middle income terms) were higher than
in villas; toilets were almost always shared with several other families,
and kitchens were sometimes shared with one or two families only.
Piped-in gas was available for stoves. The gas and electricity were
regulated by the city, and there was an occasional telephone in buildings
occupied by only two or three families. Very few bathtubs were to be
found in *conventillos,* and much of the washing was done with cold
water, outside in an open patio.

Some parts of the extensive patio running the length of the house were
sheltered. Children were usually confined to the open patio area for play,
weather permitting, and seldom went outside on the sidewalk unless
supervised by an older sibling (apparently youngsters about 10 years
old). The parents in homes I observed seemed to be quite concerned
with dressing the children well, and "proper" clothing was always worn
when children and adults left the housing area. Most of the women
worked, often as domestics in private homes, but some were employed
in factories if day care facilities were available. Commonlaw partners
seldom took the children out as a family group, although the children
might accompany the mother to her relatives' house over a holiday or
during a school vacation period. The fathers usually worked long hours
and had at least two jobs. The common-law marriage fathers were seldom
around the house, for when not working, they went out on their own.
In some extended families, with legal marriages and more living space,
the husbands had steady and better-paying jobs, including some skilled
occupations. A few such groups might have shared a *conventillo,* with
the family doing more together. Nevertheless, the parents seldom went
out together to a movie or to a friend's house for the evening. Only the
husbands seemed to go out in the evenings or on days off. Children had
little contact with their fathers.

Some of the features of the third general style of life were an ecologi-
cally separated small home or apartment, more amenities (e.g., hot water,
perhaps a telephone, occasionally an old car), and more regularized
marriage relationships, including close ties among the maternal and
paternal kin groups. A few families in this style sent their children to

private schools (often religious). Whereas in *villas miserias* and *con-centillos* one was likely to observe physically darker people—typically from Bolivia, Paraguay, or northern areas of Argentina—the lower-middle-income people found in the third group tended to be lighter-skinned immigrants or children of immigrants from European countries, particularly Italy and Spain. If the family lived in a house, it was likely to be sold, in need of repair, with many makeshift services and repairs. If the family lived in an apartment building, it would be an old, low-rise structure without an elevator; part of it (probably the kitchen and service porch) would not be entirely enclosed, thus open to the elements. The living room, if not used as a bedroom, would be reserved for special visitors and occasions and would contain seldom-used dishware and furniture.

The family might go as a group to a park or to a neighborhood movie, but the parents were not apt to go out together very often unless an in-law was living with them (a likely possibility). Occasionally the mother worked, hiring a low-paid servant to clean the house, help cook, and watch the children. The father might work for himself in a small neighborhood business, or he might have a steady job in a factory or as a municipal employee. Regular employment seemed to be common, but there was little chance of the family bettering their present circumstances. Various material goods were gradually acquired over the years, and a couple in their fifties might own a refrigerator, a stove, a sewing machine, a television set, a washing machine, a radio-phonograph set, vacuum cleaner, and a water heater.

To empasize the variability in life style that was possible within the third general living style, I have purposely used terms such as "a few," "usually," "likely," and "might" to indicate broad modalities of action. The equivocation reveals the basic distortions than can arise when we force diversities in social behavior into classes or strata that imply explicit interval scales. The appearance of hierarchy and of differences in social awareness or class consciousness were presumed in my description, but the documentation always masks subtle variations that tend to disappear when we use broad terms.

A fourth style of life would be identified by most Americans and Argentines as "middle class." A family in this group may have an older, but well-kept apartment or house, or even a newer house in one of the suburbs. The dwellings were well furnished and had many appliances, and numerous homes and apartments (with elevators) had servants' quarters. The children might be enrolled in a private school, the mother might visit the beauty parlor regularly, and the father might belong to a men's club which had occasional family functions. The children were treated to fairly elaborate birthday parties. Servants and annual vacations to the popular (and large by any standards) summer beach resort of Mar del Plata were features of this style of life. Husbands and wives were likely to go to dinner and a movie together; they entertained at home, and they maintained close family ties. The children often became university students. The family might have a car.

A fifth style of life did not differ greatly from the fourth, although as a rule one could note newer homes, more expensive appliances, more cars, higher proportion of children enrolled in private schools, more than one servant, possibly a small cottage in the country, and occasional trips abroad to Europe or the United States. There might be a small apartment owned in or near the summer resort of Mar del Plata. I think that this life style was distinguished by the extensive socializing and entertaining engaged in, and the husband's activities at a club. Furthermore, there was likely to be considerable interest in what was "fashionable," including psychotherapy and physical fitness. The people dressed in the latest fashions, and the most modern type of European and North American appliances, decor, and gadgets were likely to be found in the house or apartment.

A sixth style of life could be described as "upper class." Except for the present level of liquid assets and the repair of country and/or beach homes (e.g., at Punta del Este, Uruguay), the contrast with the preceding category might be simply a matter of larger, older homes and apartments, an "older" family name, and the like. Upper-class families possess many antiques and expensive family heirlooms. Certain traditional occupations, such as law, accounting, cattle raising, engineering, and medicine, seem to be characteristic of these families. I am familiar with only a few upper-class families, and then only superficially. My sample includes a very small number of cases, and therefore my impressions are limited.

In presenting the reader with my informal impressions of the "class structure," I hasten to add that these impressions are not reflected in the presumably objective tables presented. The "objective" measures may satisfy some researchers' and readers' conceptions of rigor, but they also conceal the kinds of impressions persons must construct imaginatively when reading tables. These impressions, like my descriptions, constitute the researcher's hidden resource for explaining what the tables "mean." The central importance of ethnographic materials is often ignored in quantitative cross-national studies. The reader will always have to formulate an opinion of what the tables could mean in terms of his own country, unless he is supplied with considerable descriptive material to serve as a basis for his independent evaluation of tables purporting to index a foreign milieu.

Characteristics of the Sample.   Table 3 indicates that the majority of the sample were born in an urbanized setting—90 (90%) of the men and 124 (81%) of the women. The determination of "urban" versus "rural" settings was not made in an exact sense, but traded on the interviewer's use of the following questions:

Place of Birth_____
Province _____
(If the place of birth is not a large city or known to the interviewer, ask:) Is (name of place) _____
located in the countryside? (Regardless of the answer, ask:) Could you tell me more about your surroundings and the house in which you lived? (Subsequent probes should include questions about the existence of paved roads, schools, hospitals, etc., in order to obtain a more detailed description of the place of birth.)

This elicitation procedure furnished an indirect basis for securing additional information about place of birth, and although the researcher went beyond the respondent's use of "rural" or "urban" by asking for details, the coding operation had to include many guesses that were occasionally buttressed by plausible supporting information. In ascertaining the ruralness or urbanness of the respondent's birthplace, it was difficult to arrive at explicit criteria for claiming that a judgment was based on independent evidence about population density and general ecological factors. The more populated cities of Argentina (called the *Litoral*) served as the principal source of comparsion for making decisions, but it was not easy to determine where the respondent had spent most of his time before adulthood and then to indicate how his background—rural or urban—had influenced his attitudes on fertility. Based on the judgments of the coders, the major part of the sample was characterized as urban. Assuming that the materials in Table 3 can be accepted at face value, it can be argued that the sample overrepresents the urban sector of the general Argentine population. Germani (1962: 220) provides a table showing that 65% of the population lived in centers of 2000 inhabitants or more in 1957, thus suggesting that our sample somewhat underrepresents respondents from a rural background.

TABLE 3.   GENERAL CHARACTERISTICS OF THE SAMPLE

Characteristics	Men	Women
Place of birth		
Rural Argentina	3	15
Urban Argentina	67	102
Semiurban Argentina	7	13
Rural area in foreign country	—	—
Urban area in foreign country	23	22
Semiurban area in foreign country	—	—
Religion		
Catholic	78	124
Protestant	4	9
Other Christian religions	2	5
Jewish	6	8
Other	—	2
None	9	4
No information	1	—
Marital status		
Common-law	1	2
Married	95	133
Separated	2	5
Divorced	1	3
Widowed	1	9
Number of unions	2	
One	93	147
Two	7	5
Three or more	—	—
Totals for each characteristic	100	152

Table 3 also reveals that the anticipated religious "preference" was largely Catholic. Primarily, married couples made up the sample, with a few divorced, separated, or second unions. The Argentine sample differed from the studies by Stycos in Puerto Rico (1955) and by Blake (1961) in Jamaica in several ways. For example, the Caribbean area samples were primarily rural in origin. The Jamaican sample was described as mainly Protestant, but the Puerto Rican group was comparable to Argentina in the number of respondents claiming to be Catholic. The Jamaican and Puerto Rican samples reveal a large number (41% for males and 23% for females in Jamaica, and 46% for both males and females in Puerto Rico) of common-law marriages as well as serial monogamy. The Argentine sample, therefore, contrasts sharply with the Jamaican and Puerto Rican studies, whereas the two Caribbean groups differ from each other only in terms of religious preference. But the design and substantive issues were quite similar for all three studies.

The Argentine sample had few common-law marriages, and few "separated" or "divorced" cases. The term "divorce" simply refers to a separation obtained under Argentine law or the laws of another country. A sort of "mail-order" divorce is possible from Mexico, and some families seek the appearance of legality offered by a divorce in Uruguay; but such activities appear to be ceremonial acts, performed chiefly for the benefit of the individuals involved, and for their friends and relatives. Neither "divorced" party is eligible for remarriage in Argentina. There are some problematic consequences of the Argentine divorce situation that should be mentioned if we are to compare the three samples. Marriages in Argentina may appear to be more stable than in Puerto Rico or Jamaica, and we could argue that stability leads to greater success in family planning efforts, assuming that the partners are in agreement about limiting the size of the family. When the highly urban character of the Argentine sample is acknowledged, the family stability argument appears to be a valid basis for suggesting that low fertility rates should be expected from this sample. But the expectation of low fertility can be explained from a different standpoint. My ethnographic impressions suggest that many marriages are stable only by appearance; given the inability to obtain a divorce, one or both spouses may live complicated lives that include other partners, while maintaining the legal and economic framework of the original marriage. Thus not only are family living patterns modified in terms of joint family activities or social activities by the partners, but sexual relationships with the legal spouse are less probable.

Only a small special sample (not reported in the tables) taken from the municipal Children's Hospital resembled the samples of Stycos and Blake. The mothers interviewed here had very low income and educational levels; there were many common-law marriages, and there tended to be a past history of rural poverty. But this special sample was not typical of Argentina's Western European type of culture, nor was it typical of the rather urban, cosmopolitan sample obtained from Buenos Aires. Most of the special sample subjects were women who were a semicaptive population at the Children's Hospital, living-in to help care for their sick infants. It was often difficult to find out whether at the time there was a male partner and whether the union was legal or common-law; it was especially difficult to make arrangements to interview the child's father, assuming he was known. How much credence could we place in the respondent's answers when she was under pressure from both hospital authorities and the interviewer (usually perceived as part of the staff) to provide "normal" answers to questions that tacitly implied a desired appearance of a "stable" union (i.e., legal marriage to the father of all her children)? The hospital records contained "double entry" answers to questions by the staff social worker, involving both oral and written gossip about the respondent's circumstances.

CHAPTER 5

METHODOLOGICAL ISSUES IN FIELD STUDIES

In studying family life, the researcher is interested in *how* members come to recognize family planning activities as relevant to their circumstances, how they become oriented to a course of action, and how they organize activities assumed to be consistent with an imagined course of action that others can recognize as meaningful. Because he can seldom be present at the actual scenes to gather verbal and nonverbal information about everyday family life, the researcher must construct enough theoretical machinery to recover the interactional features indexed by interview language. The members' use of spontaneous language categories during the interview can provide the researcher with partial depictions of the social structures. The partial depiction is a construction that can be arrived at if the interviewer is able to encourage the respondent to recreate the circumstances of the original exchanges in which routine family matters are discussed or avoided. Having an idea of how members communicate in all conversational exchanges—especially when a question–answer interview format is used—enables the researcher to ask how a particular form of communication is to be analyzed. Such analysis must recognize that communication only partially indexes different layers of meanings in the interview setting and that is aimed at reconstructing the primary source of member contact.

An investigation of human fertility must contend with issues that are typically vague, varying considerably over time. The decision-making process involved in procreation is subject to changes because of emergent day-to-day contingencies. Once family decisions are agreed on, the husband and wife may begin a process whereby "what happened" is historicized along acceptable (to others) normative lines. If decisions are reached without such historicized accounts being developed, the researcher's questions may evoke explanations suitable to the research setting. Such explanations may not reflect the original interaction, however, unless the investigator's theoretical apparatus allows for spontaneous responses and can elaborate the responses according to explicit procedures. Elaboration in this case amounts to reconstructing the everyday social organization that is presumed to be indexed by the responses.

Sociologists and some anthropologists tend to utilize kinship terms under the assumption that everybody knows the meaning of the terms within the context of a group's social organization. Such usage implies that the terms somehow stand apart from the interactional situations and conceptions that become attached to social encounters that members associate with actual kin relations. The term "mother," for example, is often invoked to convey "usual" meanings about the importance of the "mother–child" relationship; but how we would decide whether someone is a "good" mother or a "mother" in "name only" is not at all clear from the research literature on family life. Studies of fertility behavior seldom make everyday kinship relations a problematic issue for study. Ideal images of family structure are used as if such relations were "constant"; hence actual practices are often viewed as irrelevant to the problem at hand. If the researcher treats "the family" as a bounded unit, as if it possessed corporate membership qualities, he misses the significance of viewing such a structure as "a system of unbalanced dyads" (Schneider: 1965). From such a narrow perspective, one ignores the ways in which everyday meanings and behavioral realities can be at variance with members' and researchers' use of kin terms.

Thus in Argentina, because the term "divorce" means legal separation, neither party is eligible for remarriage in that country. As a consequence, many middle- and upper-income families avoid legal separation in Argentina; instead, they obtain a foreign divorce and remarry in Uruguay or Mexico. The original couple does remain legally married, but now there are different "families," in which visiting rights preserve consanguineous relations for children, yet affinal relations follow unclear rules depending on parental friendships. Confusion regarding terminology can occur for both children and parents. To illustrate some related problems I encountered in my research, I turn to some impressionistic materials on a few families.

Substantive Issues and Methodological Consequences.   From the research experiences of the Argentine study I learned that trying to understand the social context of the family at the time of the first contact is like walking into a theater in the middle of an unknown motion picture and trying to decide what is going on.

Two general problems must be disentangled here: (a) the substantive problem of the circumstances the interviewer might walk into when he first rings the doorbell (e.g., a recurrent family argument about the husband's infidelity or lack of interest in the wife and children, negotiations for a divorce, worry about an unemployed husband, or problems caused by a sick child, that seem to make everyone and everything appear depressing to the family members), and (b) the basic research problem of identifying language and interactional categories that alert the researcher to possible clues of how family interaction is motivated. The language used, which presumably reflects specific structural features of the society, can also suggest the routine grounds for decision-making during family interaction. The researcher must know something of (b) in order to address the problems in (a).

If the researcher is committed to principles more rigorous than those of a mechanical role theory that views commonsense meanings as obvious, he must specify the typical categories used by family members for depicting their problems to one another *and* to the researcher. Hence interview material can be deceptive unless the researcher is prepared to advance conjectures regarding how the interview talk employed by the respondent reveals specifiable conceptions of family life and of the respondent's everyday environment. Specifically, what is typical for the respondent? What is typical and acceptable conduct for husbands? for children? What sorts of boundary conditions define the wife's notion of male adequacy vis-à-vis the husband's occupational activities, his income, his attention to her, their sexual relations, the desirability of children, the number of children desired, and so forth? What are "justifiable" grounds for being "angry," obtaining a divorce, starting an argument, "making up," or demanding an apology? The everyday meanings employed by family members for making sense of their relationships help to sustain the family as a self-regulating unit for routinely handling the daily problems of living at close quarters. This system of interaction should not be detached from the larger context within which issues about family planning and fertility are related to problems of population growth and economic development. To ignore such connections is to ignore the way patterns of social process interface with the aggregated statistical outcomes we label structural effects at the demographic level of analysis.

The respondent's views (or lack of them) can be effectively concealed in many ways during an interview, and space does not permit a detailed catalog of such contingencies. Briefly, they include the relationship between interviewer and respondent, the current or persistent family circumstances that seem to overshadow the topics projected by the questionnaire or interview schedule, ignorance of the topics, and indifference to the topics. The descriptions that follow are intended to illustrate some of the ethnographic settings encountered in a few families I visited frequently.

FAMILY A. This low-income family—parents and their two children—lived in a poor suburb of Buenos Aires. Their three room house was built by the husband, who was employed as a traffic policeman in a nearby suburb and supplemented his income with odd jobs such as cooking barbecues at a private club. (The situation was similar to that of many Argentine families, since municipal, state, or federal jobs did not pay enough to support them during inflationary times, and second jobs were routine for the breadwinners.) The wife was arthritic at 37 and required the help of her husband to complete the daily tasks of living under difficult circumstances. The youngest child, a girl of 3, had been ill with what a physician had defined as psychologically induced *petit mal* seizures. The husband frequently became very angry when the girl fell during a seizure. His "explosions" revolved around her illness, the cost of living and inflation, and the problems of maintaining the household.

It was difficult to induce the wife to discuss in depth any of the questions dealing with fertility; she appeared to be both ignorant of the issues and indifferent to my many probes, yet concerned that she was probably not "helping" me. She was quite willing to discuss family planning and the use of contraceptives, although she had little to say about these activities, and she did not hesitate to answer that she and her husband engaged in sexual intercourse two or three times a week—adding that she saw little choice but to comply with his demands, lest he look elsewhere. Her responses to my questions suggested that she wanted two boys and two girls, but she noted that her physical condition would make it difficult. She then revealed that the husband preferred no children, that she was afraid to use contraceptives, that they were too costly, and that the husband was the one who sought to prevent pregnancies. The wife indicated that the husband had wanted her to abort the second child and that a physician had given her some injections for that purpose, but without success. Her responses suggested that the expressed wishes of the husband were adequate grounds for action, but she seemed interested in communicating her differences of opinion.

The husband, on the other hand, seemed to enjoy discussing some questions merely as a way of digressing from the issue and taking advantage of a captive audience (the interviewer). He truncated his remarks about family planning and fertility, however, indicating that times were "too hard" for thinking about additional children. His wife seldom left the house, nor was she active in political or religious affairs, although she had once been a very active supporter of Perón. The Argentine climate and the general atmosphere of the house made interviewing difficult; it was exceptionally hot and humid and there seemed to be thousands of flies everywhere. The children fought often, the wife frequently continued her work while answering questions, and many responses suggested that she did not welcome probing questions in most of the areas I brought up. Both parents appeared reluctant to participate in the interview, yet they seemed quite interested in continuing general conversation and insisted that I have more tea or another drink. It was necessary for me to explain each question to both the husband and the wife after presenting it, to clarify the question's intended meaning.

I visited the home often during a period of several months, went out for a beer with the husband, and met the wife and the epileptic child at the children's hospital to help them obtain additional medical care— yet the questions I posed seemed to be inappropriate, misunderstood. The questions opened up areas that seemed to be strange because they apparently bore no relevance to the family's everyday problems. It was difficult to press either parent to express how deeply each one felt about having more children or to what lengths the couple would go to prevent more children. The wife kept saying "Isn't that so?" after her responses, as if to inquire whether she had answered properly, or to avoid a probing comeback by the interviewer. Both spouses indicated that life before marriage had been more exciting and had involved more social activities and more money, whereas their present situation permitted little or nothing in the way of entertaining, outings, or material possessions. The husband seemed to want to put me off by responding, "We talk about it, we talk about it," or "Things are the same, the same, it's all the same, it's all the same," implying that he was not interested in answering such questions but did not want to be rude to me.

FAMILY B. This young couple (husband 23, wife 21) lived with the woman's parents in a middle-income area. They had one child, 8 months old. Only the wife completed an interview. I encountered the husband one morning when he was going to work, but because of his (apparently) odd working hours as an appliance repairman, I was unable to arrange a second meeting with him after many attempts and after completing an initial part of the schedule. I spoke to the husband on three separate occasions—while he was busy repairing his car, just as he was to leave for work, and shortly after he returned from work for lunch. There was a telephone in the house, making it possible to communicate with the family many times, and although the response always appeared to be friendly, it was difficult to know whether they were intentionally avoiding me. The wife's answers were polite and apparently based on complete comprehension of the material, but almost always they were expressed in quick, short phrases, frequently with a "no" that seemed quite final. She appeared anxious throughout the interview, sitting on the edge of the chair, and often looking to see how far away her mother was. I became uneasy and continually explained the study to her, in an attempt to set us both at ease. She had been trained to teach elementary school but had become pregnant before beginning to work full time. Both she and her husband had wanted the first child immediately, but she wanted to wait until the present child was older before having another. She stated that three children, spaced two years apart, was an ideal family size. She seemed to be aware of contraceptive devices but kept avoiding any commitment regarding use of them, saying that her husband had been using condoms since the baby's birth. The woman gave a picture of comfortable living and an active social life but acknowledged that "life was hard" because of inflation and political instability. It was difficult to probe any area to establish a wider family context, and I stopped asking questions on some subjects because of the woman's evident anxiety and her curt, somewhat frightened "no's." Her responses were short and concise, but occasionally she denied having an opinion, which I interpreted as her way of forestalling further comments.

It would not be difficult to code the information provided by families A and B, perhaps finishing with similar classifications for attitudes on family planning and the control of family size. It would be easy to find a basis for justifying the use of a standard code, under the assumption that the questions and answers addressed the same topics and were understood by respondents in identical ways. But the standard questions impinged on different environments. Even if the reader questioned the interviewer's skills, he would have to admit that standard coding procedures fail to clarify the means by which the researcher's tables eliminate the contingencies generated by many factors—including the variations in interviewer success with the respondent, the family setting that forms part of what is expected as an answer, and the use of truncated or negative responses, which obscure the possible alternative meanings that can be attributed to the utterances. The wife of family B, therefore, is of interest precisely because it would be easy to ignore the setting and her truncated, managed responses, proceeding to code the answers as though they had the same significance as the responses given by the husband and wife of family A. Separating the families by social class does not resolve the basic problem of finding the meaning of the questions as they are administered in particular social settings by specific interviewers.

FAMILY C. A 60-year-old widow lived alone in an old house in a working-class suburb and supported herself by selling roosters and working a small garden. Her husband had been killed by an automobile. The Spanish-born respondent described her life as miserable from the day her mother had died, leaving the child of 7 to grow up in a foster home with a foster mother whom she hated and who hated her. She married her husband because he seemed like a decent person and a good provider, was about to buy her present house, and had a skill. They were married young (she was 20, he was 24) and they both worked hard making bricks in their back yard. The husband treated her badly soon after the marriage and was always out of the house when not working.

The couple had one daughter, and although the wife wanted more children, she was unable to have them for "physical reasons," which the interviewer interpreted as physiological problems. When the daughter reached 11 or 12 years of age, the woman's neighbors began to tell her that her husband was having sexual relations with the girl. She did not believe the stories until she realized that her husband was keeping their daughter home from school and sending the respondent away on errands, to be with the child more often. The wife stopped having sexual relations with her husband after that. Her husband treated her very badly, to the point of using his mother's name on official forms, thus making it difficult for her to claim his retirement pay. She evaded questions about the use of contraceptives, saying there were "natural ways" of preventing children and that one could not ignore one's religion in such matters. Yet she felt that it was best not to have more children than one could raise adequately, feed properly, educate, and the like. She cried at different points in the interview, lamenting her miserable life, her lack of education, and her lack of knowledge—even of the pretty parts of Buenos Aires which she had never been able to visit. It was difficult for the interviewer to probe her answers because they were circuitous and guarded.

The need to decide how to treat such information, which becomes historicized or retrospective because of present conditions, raises the question of whether only women of childbearing age should be included in a fertility study. We must determine how the respondent, at any age, reconstructs his or her past views for the interview in light of present circumstances, and how the future (e.g., family planning) is affected in a similar fashion when it is realized that any number of changes could occur to change any existing plans. Therefore, if we code the responses of the older woman in family C with standard rules that would be used for families A and B, there is no way of allowing for the temporal reconstruction inherent in the respondents' notions of family planning, sexual relations, use of contraceptives, ideas about marital happiness, and the like.

FAMILY D.   This lower-middle-income family lived in a house built by the husband in an upper-middle income area; there were three boys, ages 8, 16, and 18. During the marriage, the husband and wife have disagreed about the number of children they should have. The wife has had four abortions. The woman had wanted to use contraceptives but believed that existing methods such as the diaphragm or the coil would cause cancer. The husband had used condoms sporadically but tended to rely on the withdrawal procedure. He seemed indifferent to the consequences of not always being careful, although he commented that too many children make the woman's job difficult and increase the husband's responsibility for support. The husband's responses did not indicate any concern with sexual relations, family planning, and the use of contraceptives; his answers, always direct and short, gave me the impression that he would rather discuss more important problems such as finding work or building a house in the country to get away from the city. The wife's remarks on the use of contraceptives, family planning, and sexual relations contrasted sharply because he had always regarded sexual relations as a problem in and of itself. She feared the use of the diaphragm and the coil, although she wanted to prevent future pregnancies, and she felt that two children would have been the ideal size but had borne the third in hopes of having a girl. The husband, who had not wanted the third child, decided that he wanted more after the baby arrived. The husband liked boys because they could help him with his work. The woman stated flatly that she often went to bed early, pretending to be asleep or feigning a headache or other minor discomfort to avoid sexual activity. She lived in terror of becoming pregnant again and felt that her husband did not control himself adequately to prevent another pregnancy. She would have been happier if the risk of pregnancy were eliminated from their marriage.

Although the woman appeared to be quite tense and frequently remarked about her "nervousness," the husband seemed quite cheerful and outgoing. According to the wife, the husband preferred staying home and watching television or going to the country to work on the other house he was building, to going out to the movies or to downtown Buenos Aires. The husband was born in Italy and had come to Argentina when he was 12; the wife's family was Italian, but she was born in Argentina. She regarded her husband, as an "old fashioned" immigrant, and felt that she was a "modern" American. (Here "American" is used in the same sense that it is used in the United States to distinguish between "old country" and up-to-date "American" ways of living.) The husband believed that his life should be oriented around his work and that the wife should simply cook, clean, and be accessible in bed. The woman felt that one should try to increase the children's chances of getting ahead in the world by giving them more schooling opportunities rather than by having them work at the same occupation as the father, and that parents should be close to their children and not treat them as "workers." The woman believed that the couple should have more social life, read more, and become more active politically. She was an ardent supporter of Perón; he was not. She gave me a copy of one of Perón's books and told me how she used to light candles for "Evita" [Perón] but was afraid the police would find out and cause trouble. She indicated that the couple seldom talked about family planning and only managed to discuss financial problems at bedtime. Her husband casually stated that they discussed "many things."

I spent many afternoons and weekends with this family and felt that most of the time the husband and wife were talking past each other. They often started arguments in my presence, and when the wife said, for example, "See how he is," he shrugged his shoulders and said "Women are always getting excited about the unimportant things." For the wife, the interviewer represented a professional audience to whom she could confide problems that could not be discussed with others. She did not like her husband's family and had few friends of her own. She saw the interviewer as a person with expert training who would understand her predicament. It would be difficult to say whether another interviewer would have encountered the same reception, since in my case there was an important added ingredient: I had helped the wife obtain medical advice at the Childrens' Hospital, where I was conducting another study. She also asked me for advice about contraceptive devices and about her youngest child. I did not hesitate to give advice, but only after the formal interviewing was completed.

FAMILY E. Legally separated from her husband according to Argentine law, the woman lived with two sons and one daughter in a modest, well-furnished house in a middle-income suburb. She had two other daughters who were married. Her former husband, a professional man, "married" his assistant after the legal separation. During her marriage the respondent had lived an upper-class existence in one of Buenos Aires' most fashionable districts, there had been a large house with many servants, many parties, a summer home, and the like. After the separation her life had become difficult and embittered because she could not live as before and give her children what she felt they deserved. She described her younger years in glowing terms, her marriage and life with the children's father as proper, exciting, and fashionable. She had always been a staunch Catholic, was opposed to the legal separation (and was still bewildered by it), and would never use contraceptives (nor would her husband), affirming that all children that happened to be born would be welcome. She noted that she and her husband had not discussed sexual activities or family planning because they believed that such topics were "natural" and simply were to be taken for granted. Her children—ages 20, 22, 25, 27, and 30—had been caught in the middle of this downward mobile experience and had been obliged to modify their future occupational aspirations and marriage plans.

This woman's answers were always direct; she was always quite poised when responding, and although apparently surprised by the questions on the use of contraceptives, she did not evade them. She did exhibit reticence in discussing frequency of intercourse, preferring to state that she and her husband always "got along" with each other privately. Then she would launch into a somewhat bitter commentary on "that woman" who had ruined everything for her. Her interpretation of questions about sexual relations and the use of contraceptives cannot be taken literally, because she made it clear that her sexual relations were no one else's business. Moreover, she did not feel qualified to discuss contraceptives, since she said that she knew nothing about their availability or use and did not care to know, claiming that such devices were never relevant to her life. This woman seemed to follow an orthodox Catholic religious view of family planning but did not seem to be offended by the questions. She was evidently quite happy to speak to someone about her life circumstances and appeared to brighten considerably when describing what for her had been a "glorious" past. Coffee and cookies were served during each of several visits, and the respondent made every attempt to adjust her schedule to that of the interviewer. Yet in spite of all the appearances of excellent rapport, responses were managed, truncated, or avoided areas that she considered to be "private."

I chose to discuss these five families on ad hoc grounds because they were known to me; indeed I had interviewed them all, except family C. An attempt to become acquainted with the general family context by way of open-ended questions and extensive probes gave the researcher a backdrop against which questions could be interpreted. Cross-tabulation and the construction of scales generate meaning structures, as imposed by the method of analysis. Furthermore, such procedures do not allow the investigator to understand the respondents' utterances as employed and intended within the socially organized context of the family interviewed, nor do they account for the relationship of the interviewer and respondent.

The Research Strategy.   In my Argentine study I sought to utilize the general framework of a survey design, featuring a small sample and with open-ended questions, which were designed to provide the respondent with a minimal definition of the problem at hand. Rather than assume that the actor was familiar with the intent of a question, I employed the question as an initial thrust, to test the respondent's perception of what was going on in the interview situation and to give some direction to my intentions in interviewing. The interviewers were instructed to allow the respondent to use his or her own words, encouraging free association. A few general questions were employed to elicit spontaneous remarks about problems of routine family life and particularly any problem in the husband–wife relationship. Although essentially a replication of work done by Blake in Jamaica (1961), the present study is different in that the interviewers were told the following: (*a*) unremarkable or evasive answers given in response to standardized questions should be followed by probes aimed at encouraging the respondent to mention family problems spontaneously in the course of the interview, (*b*) it was important to discover linkages or discrepancies between what was being asked and answered formally and what might be revealed by further probing and by spontaneous remarks from the subject during the course of the interview, and (c) a description of the social context of the interview, both initially and as conditions changed, should be included to enable the interviewer to make sense of the respondent's utterances. The interviewers received extra pay for writing down postinterview descriptions of the general atmosphere of the session; problems they had experienced with respect to general or particular questions; their feelings about whether the subject had been lying, evading the issue, or had not understood the question; and problems in their relationship with the respondent.

The methodological strategy was dictated by theoretical assumptions about the nature of family life. The interviewer has no way of knowing what manner of family predicaments he will encounter. In addition to the suspicion of strangers endemic to very large metropolitan areas, the political situation in Buenos Aires and Argentina in general was rather unstable; thus many interviewers were taken for municipal or federal officials interested in making trouble for the respondents. Even when there is apparent readiness by respondents to submit to the interview, however, we have no guarantee that the subjects will pose no objections to the interview, or that we are going to be able to successfully question people about matters social scientists are often reluctant to probe; we cannot conclude that the material obtained is a valid indication of everyday practice and belief.

I assumed that the most important factor in an interview was the social relationship between the interviewer and the respondent during the course of the interaction. I also believed that two or more visits would be necessary to lead to fruitful probing and spontaneous remarks about family routines and problems. Hence the interviewers were told to begin with the part of the schedule that involved seemingly objective material, and to seek a second or third interview to cover areas that were considered to be delicate and yet quite possibly revelatory about persistent problems of family life. Better relations were often established because many appointments had to be made and remade. The frequent contact enabled us to become acquainted with our subjects long before we arrived at the more delicate or difficult questions. There were times, of course, when the interviewer seemed to strike precisely the right note on the initial encounter, but such occasions were not typical. Each interview proved to be a "problem" in itself, and each had to be negotiated at every step.

The problems we label methodological are not merely "technical" obstacles to "ideal" interviewing; they are natural and inevitable components of field research. The probing and the spontaneous qualitative materials are not merely supplements to the "objective" quantitative data we obtain from surveys, census reports, and vital statistic reports, in which the qualitative material is seen as problematic because of the difficulties in coding the information. We are enabled to assign meaning to presumed objective information by virtue of the elicitation of qualitative material and the constructed meanings that are attached to it.

The negotiated character of field research, therefore, is itself a documentation of the structure of social interaction—that is, the structure of social interaction is reflected by such factors as the difficulties inherent in negotiating the first appointment and each stage of the interview, the various social types of actors encountered, the resistances to specific questions or blocs of questions, the need to convince the respondent to complete the interview, and the problem of motivating the interviewer to regard each interview as an important case.

Throughout the field research I assumed that the choice of interviewers, like the use of "stooges" in experimental research (Leik 1965) is subject to limited control. Therefore, some way of accounting for the influence of the interviewer's presence on what pass as "data" became a critical part of the reported "findings."

The "impact" of two sets of actors—the interviewers and the subjects—can be known only after the completion of the interview unless partial control is possible. Consider the following strategy: interviewers were instructed to terminate the first visit after the "objective" section (questions about age, sex, education, income, etc.) was completed if they felt that they could not get along with the subject or if they felt uncomfortable with the household or with one or both spouses. In consultation with the principal investigator, the interviewer then tried to give enough pertinent information about the respondent to permit the selection of another interviewer who might work better with the social type characterization reported by the unsuccessful worker. The mesh between interviewer and respondent could never be perfect, even under the best procedures available. Therefore, details about recurrent problems were essential if the researcher were to evaluate adequately the influence of the communication network that was developed between interviewer and respondent on questions, responses, and outcomes labeled as data. The researcher discussed this problem of mesh, to make it easy for the interviewer to admit to such problems as a natural part of the research situation. Many interviewers were concerned lest they lose interviews, hence diminish the amount of money they would earn. Therefore, I allowed for another possibility: an interviewer who lost an interview could spend an equivalent amount of time, with adequate compensation (agreed in advance), writing about the problems he had encountered with the respondent—for example, the usefulness or uselessness of the questions, the communication problems, the perceived social difference in background that might have hindered the interview, deliberate withholding of information, and so forth.

Five general types of respondents seemed to emerge: (a) those who refused to begin an interview; (b) those who consented to begin the interview but stopped before completion (among these were a few cases in which one spouse was interviewed and the other refused during some part of the session) ; (c) respondents who made remarks that the interviewer judged to be "honest" but truncated in terms of the details and subtleties given, such that the informational content appeared to be carefully monitored throughout; (d) those whose answers were described by the interviewer as "sincere" or "honest" at times, and "evasive" or "contrived" at other times, although all the answers seemed to be truncated and carefully monitored; and (e) interviewees who appeared to be "sincere" in giving most answers in depth with little or no encouragement, thus providing many spontaneous reactions to questions and independent remarks about their responses to the standard questions or probes. All interviews included occasions of the respondent apparently being ignorant of the practice or circumstances referred to by the questions, or not sure what was intended by the question or explanation given by the interviewer. Furthermore, the foregoing descriptions are ideal-typical—no case fitted a category perfectly. For example, some refusals were preceded by as much as three hours of discussion, wine drinking, and friendly conversation.

Interviewers were instructed first to present the question in the standardized way, as it appeared on the written schedule. If the subject did not appear to comprehend the question, this impression was to be noted before the interviewer attempted to explain what *was* intended. Thus it was assumed that in addition to the ignorance factor, which could be operating at any stage of the interview, there is also the following linguistic problem—that of not being able to formulate question in such a way that a wide spectrum of the population could interpret its intended meaning in identical ways.

The interviewer–respondent mesh carries still another assumption—namely, that each person employs linguistic styles and other socially relevant body movements, gestures, or facial expressions that communicate a variety of meanings and bits of information about social character, social background, political views, and the like. Such communication may serve to inhibit or to facilitate the interview per se as a comfortable social exchange. For example, it may influence the duration of the interview as each party seeks to bargain in implicit terms about what will be tolerated, and as each seeks to convey or to blur an image of himself, his relative interest in the other as a person, and so on.

The extent to which the interviewer–respondent mesh can be termed "successful," "tolerable," or a "failure" requires an indication of how the interviewer decided that he or she had successfully communicated with the respondent. Many interviewers might be afraid to admit failure to establish good relations with the respondent or to note that the information obtained was inadequate in places. Although I employed a few weak interviewers, the three women who did most of the interviewing not only had considerable experience, but were not afraid to admit to problems; moreover, they called me frequently to consult about the way in which particular exchanges were unfolding.

Maintaining a constant, high motivational level when interviewing intensively over time is difficult work. After a number of interviews it is easy to develop a perfunctory routine for going through the questions. Many researchers are hard put to keep interest high over time. I found that constant communication with the interviewers throughout the study was critical for motivating them to share special and routine problems about each case. Inasmuch as I was also doing interviews, it was easy to refer to my own difficulties and to obtain immediate responses from the interviewers about their problems. Whenever possible, I sought to tape record or take detailed notes on exchanges with interviewers about particular cases and the problems that emerged. We reviewed the cases at the time when the interviewers were paid. When there seemed to be an unusual number of rejections or high resistance in a district, a special strategy was planned for learning more about the difficulties. One such occasion resulted in a plan that offered payment to the prospective interviewee and a kind of saturation schedule of interviews in the area. This tactic led to the discovery of a "witch"—according to the families refusing to be interviewed, the accused woman had told the neighborhood that they would become victims of a hex if they participated. Our presence was described as a bad omen for the area.

While the concrete problems described are common to field research, the type of interviewing conducted was intended as an alternative strategy to the conventional survey. Specifically, I sought to avoid the use of fixed-choice questions couched in language that is assumed to be universally understood in identical ways by a representative sample of the population. Instead, I stressed the following:

1. The routine basis for making sense of an utterance carries with it a general social context of unstated meanings. These unstated meanings enable the participants to decode and encode verbal and nonverbal messages.

2. In the Spanish language the structural distinctions between the familiar and polite forms of grammatical usage make differences in verbal exchanges fairly obvious. The language style employed provides specific background expectancies that are helpful to the participants in becoming oriented to each other.

3. The routine grounds for making sense of communication rely on tacit meanings in the language of everyday life and are not subject to verification unless the interviewer is willing to risk embarrassing or annoying the respondent. Hence probes that keep pressing the respondent (e.g., "Could you tell me more about that?" "Could you explain that a little more?" "How's that?") are potentially useful but may lead to an abrupt termination of the interview. Such probes, however, can clarify some of the vague or taken-for-granted terms and phrases that the respondent characteristically uses as a competent member of the society.

4. The actor's remarks in the interview, even when termed "spontaneous," are often the product of a carefully monitored kind of presentation, save, perhaps, under extreme circumstances such as uncontrolled rage or excitement. Open-ended questions posed by the researcher are also likely to be carefully monitored by the respondent. Therefore, the content of the respondent's communication cannot be divorced from such factors as choice of words, tone of voice, gestures, and facial expressions.

5. Both the interviewer and the respondent are likely to make similar attempts to appear "convincing" to each other, while minimizing remarks that may disturb the situation. Each will seek to "psych out" what the other intends by certain phrases, gestures, or voice intonations, in an effort to categorize better the utterances to which each is exposed. Therefore, sociological notions of status and role expectations cannot be invoked to explain such properties of communication. The researcher cannot justify his questions (open or fixed-choice in construction) unless he is prepared to indicate how the respondent's answers are managed products that are negotiated with the interviewer over the course of the interview.

Shortly before the study in Argentina terminated, another research group conducted a sample survey on fertility and family planning with fixed-choice questions. The two studies contained a partial overlap in the interviewers employed. The questionnarie of the second study could be completed in approximately 45 to 60 minutes, yet it covered essentially the same material of my original interview schedule. The following paragraphs summarized the problems of the second survey.

The fixed-choice questionnaire discouraged or simply cut off spontaneous comments by the respondent. Problems of ignorance or misunderstanding the questions often led to "no" responses or to what appeared to be arbitrary choices.

The questions permitted the respondent to give little information about family organization except in abbreviated form.

The attitudinal questions did not permit any independent evaluation by the interviewer regarding the evasiveness or "honesty" of the respondent, the general social context of the interview, and similar factors.

Clarifying exchanges between the respondent and interviewer were discouraged; even when they occurred, they seldom appeared on the questionnaire. Many times the interviewer felt impelled or was requested to "educate" the respondents vis-à-vis the intent of a question; but the report did not indicate how the interviewer handled the situation.

The interviewer frequently had to explain a question and then try to interpret or improvise the respondent's answer by assigning it to one of the choices available. Both the respondent's interpretation and his response were managed. Furthermore, the interviewer's marking of a particular response category was based on a more extensive interpretation of the respondent's answer than the questionnaire itself permitted.

The fixed-choice questionnaire eliminated the need for the interviewer to employ commonsense knowledge and reasoning in obtaining the material. Methodologically, the problematic features of the interview itself were removed by the very nature of the instrument. The instructions to repeat each question three times and then proceed, disallowed the possibility of including interviewer impressions and remarks about his or her doubts about answers, the respondent's observations about what was not understood, or other comments suggesting the irrelevance of differential meaning of the questions.

In the next two chapters I attempt to document in more detail the problems raised here, while addressing substantive issues about Argentine fertility behavior and family organization.

CHAPTER 6

THE METHODOLOGICAL CONTEXT

OF SUBSTANTIVE ISSUES IN FERTILITY

Questionnaire studies usually seek information on a variety of conditions affecting fertility behavior. These conditions include finding a relationship between knowledge or opinions of contraceptives and their use, or the use of abortions, as well as the cost to the respondent of using contraceptives or obtaining an abortion, attitudes about family size and the spacing of children, premarital sexual activities, age at marriage, and the duration of any sexual union. Researchers have identified other variables, of course, but the preceding conditions are often central to studies of fertility behavior.

In this chapter I want to raise the following issues:

1. How are data gathered and interpreted to supply the researcher with evidence for his claim that the variables, just named, influence fertility behavior?

2. How might we describe traditional methods and inferences, which are derived from interview and questionnaire materials, in a different way, thus arriving at different substantive theories and findings?

I propose treating the methods, data, and findings as problematic historicized activities. This approach contrasts with the interpreted outcomes of traditional studies which are never in doubt because normative constraints will ensure or guarantee appropriate substantive conclusions. By "appropriate" I mean that a normatively acceptable explanation will be forthcoming (e.g., "Women desire few children but are not socially and psychologically prepared to prevent higher fertility outcomes," or "The lower the socioeconomic status of the family, the higher the fertility rate"). The researcher's reconstruction of the data-gathering process and the data-coding processes obscures the commonsense views of the respondents and the interviewers and coders, and "surprises" occur only within the limits imposed by the variables designated as relevant to the questions asked of respondents.

Sexual Unions as a Topic. One practical problem of studying sexual unions lies in the assumption that group members are concerned with the prevention of premarital sexual activity and that this member preoccupation is an important resource for learning about sexual norms.

Researchers ask questions about sexual unions because a population's fertility rate can be affected by early or late unions. Furthermore, if early unions are preceded by considerable premarital sexual relations, we might expect increased fertility because of consensual unions and illegitimate births, particularly if there is minimal use of contraceptives and abortions in the population studied. Researchers ask questions intended to elicit information about age at marriage and about the respondent's idea of an "ideal" age for marriage. When the latter type of information is linked to informants' remarks about sexual promiscuity among males and females, premarital sex relations, and the use of contraceptives and abortions, inferences are drawn about the possibilities of higher or lower fertility rates. It is possible to argue that whereas high fertility exists, it does not reflect the informants' desires about family size but, instead, their inability to convert their attitudes into action (e.g., because of ignorance of sexual practices and contraceptives; cultural beliefs about the desirability of children, particularly among males; fear of never being married; or lack of financial resources leading to dependence on one or more consensual partners). Or, it could be argued that consensual unions may lead to maximum fertility in one setting and less than maximum fertility in another, because of the instability of the union.

All field studies employ elicitation procedures to gather materials that can be converted into data about conditions affecting fertility. The researcher then speculates about the antecedent behavioral activities that could have produced the questionnaire responses from which inferences are to be made about social structure and fertility rates. In the present study I tried to pose questions that were similar to those of Stycos (1955) and Blake (1961), while seeking to clarify carefully some of the behavioral sequences presupposed by the researcher's questions and the respondents' answers. I was not very successful in many cases because the ways in which the questions were posed allowed respondents to condense their answers about the sequence of events and/or the details of encounters during courtship or during any relationship leading to sexual unions. These problems are discussed below.

An examination of Table 1 reveals that most of the families or individuals (approximately 75%) reported a courtship longer than one year. The information in Table 1 tells nothing about the practical circumstances surrounding the duration of the engagement period, nor about condtions that would increase or decrease the possibilities of having children. We can obtain information indirectly on these contingencies, and on the researcher's necessary speculations about them and the findings claimed, by considering actual cases.

To illustrate the researcher's reconstruction of the data-gathering process, I arbitrarily selected the first two completed interviews that satified the coding categories used in the original questionnaire. The first case to be described was the interviewer's first assignment, and she claimed to have been somewhat nervous about interviewing the older couple in question—the wife was 69, the husband was 68, and they had met when they were 43 and 42, respectively. The woman had worked as a chef for some 23 years until she married. She had never been pregnant. Her husband had four children from a previous marriage. When asked a standard question about the age at which she began to go out with young men to the movies, for a walk, or to a dance, she replied, "18 years." The wife claimed to have had only one boyfriend, who visited her at home twice a week. She described her parents indirectly while answering a

TABLE 1.   DURATION OF ENGAGEMENT PRIOR TO PRESENT MARRIAGE[a]

Duration of Engagement	Frequency
Less than six months	12
Six months to one year	29
One to two years	45
More than two years	80
No information	4
Total	170

[a] The couple or spouse that answered the question formed the basis for tabulating the results. No serious disagreements occurred between spouses when both were interviewed, but when only one spouse was interviewed, the response was used for the couple without further verification.

question about her mother's reaction to the boyfriend. (The Spanish version of the following interchanges is in the Appendix at the end of the chapter.)

1. INTERVIEWER. What did he do?
   RESPONDENT. I would receive him in my house, he would come in the early evening two times a week. My parents were very (sensitive) "delicate." (FA 7 MU 1-19;o)

I assumed that the woman was explaining the "two times a week" with her remark about how "delicate" her parents were, suggesting that they would only tolerate two visits a week. The implication was that the parents were strict and perhaps made the possibility of premarital intercourse unlikely. She was subsequently asked the following question:

2. INTERVIEWER. How frequently would you see each other? Where?
   RESPONDENT. Every 15 or 20 days because the parents were "delicate," they did not want us to see each other every day. (FA 7 MU 1-19;w)

The second remark appeared to have contradicted the earlier statement that the boyfriend had visited twice a week. However, she repeated the reference to the parents as "delicate." In the next question the respondent was asked whether this was the first man with whom she had sexual relations; the answer was negative, implying he was her first boyfriend but not her first sexual contact. The second part of the question was a probe and produced in response:

3. INTERVIEWER. Could you tell me something more about this? [If this was the first man with whom she had sexual relations?]
   RESPONDENT. My present husband wants to have relations every four days, but he can't and becomes very nervous. He attempts it (sexual relations) when he is well but not when he is angry. He then bangs (himself, his head) against the wall. (FA 7 MU 1-21;y)

By using open-ended questions we attempted to generate details and broad conceptions about everyday family life in the hope of eliciting as much ethnographic background as possible, to offset the static question–answer format. Since the woman's remark did not appear to be a response to the probe, we might speculate along one or any number of the following lines: that she did not have anything to report about the first man she had dated socially, that she did not want to bring up the affair again, that her present marriage was felt to be more "interesting" for the interviewer, that her remarks were intended to open up a more serious problem than the original question and probe touched on, or that she viewed the questions as invitations or excuses for getting at her present circumstances.

Should we treat the woman's response as an answer to a question she had perceived in a facial expression or thought she had heard, although it was not expressed orally by the interviewer? The issue is a difficult one: an interrogative statement can provide the basis for a declarative response that may range from being called an "answer" to the question, to being a way of introducing a different topic, to being an attempt to avoid a topic. Interviewer and respondent must engage in interpretive work in deciding whether a response is "appropriate" and whether it can both "satisfy" the interviewer and "protect" or communicate particular ideas held by the respondent. Yet this interpretive work is neither part of the demographer's or sociologist's theory, nor is it acknowledged as basic for making such methods work and for interpreting the findings.

People engaged in conversation draw on particulars located in the setting to represent more elaborate conceptions about their own motives, their credentials, their sincerity, their social relationships with each other, their biographical histories (including age, sex, and communicative competence), as well as the relevance of a particular occasion to what is said and not said, and the consequences for accounts about past and future encounters that can be elaborated indefinitely.

Before I began an interview and while I was locating the house in a specific neighborhood, I reflected on the neighborhood, the exterior of the house, my initial perception of the respondent, the kind of talk preceding the start of formal questions, and so forth. As the exchange unfolded, I used terms I hoped would be relevant to the respondent, while simultaneously using these terms to further index the immediate scene. These thoughts and terms became embedded in my memory of the event and were employed in subsequent oral and nonoral particulars in my interpretation and description of the materials. My use of terms was designed to invite the respondent to relate her experiences by reference to the same terms, yet introducing her own langauge, too. As the interview schedule proceeded, we both infused our talk with each other's terms, which thus became particulars indexing larger horizons of meaning both within and external to the exchange. The real time of the question–answer format was continuously interlaced with the respondent's and my own inner-time conceptions of past encounters and the interview scene. It was therefore difficult to think of each question as a distinct, normative topicalizer that bounded its own referents and those of the respondent. The researcher's use of normal interrogative statements provides both the interviewer and respondent with a ready-made basis for presuming "correct" or "appropriate" questions and answers.

A verbatim transcript does not settle the issue created when there is an apparent shift in topic in response to the probe "Could you tell me something more about this?" (FA 7 MU 1-19;y), for there is no way to justify the response by a strict reference to previous questions as stimuli. The question–answer (stimulus–response) format can be misleading. Interviewer and respondent are presumed to process the questions and answers in similar ways: both are coding bundles of information that are not being recorded verbatim, yet these bundles of information are being used to initiate questions and formulate probes (by the interviewer) and to interpret questions and formulate answers (by the respondent). The verbatim exchange and the information not verbalized but nevertheless, assumed to be operative, presuppose considerably more than can be explained by reference to linguistic theory (e.g., they presuppose the factors noted earlier of age, sex, credentials, sincerity, social relationships, etc.). Each bit of information recognized explicitly or tacitly is a particular embedded in the scene (hence perhaps irrelevant in other settings), and it in turn can serve as an index for the larger expressions as the dialogue continues. Each participant negotiates his interpretation of the setting according to the organization of personal experiences, while the coder and the research analyst organize the verbatim transcript (questionnaire) as an orderly real-time sequence of "appropriate" questions and answers.

The Condensed Structure of Elicited Events. Let us return to our discussion of the woman who responded to a probe about sexual relations with her first boyfriend by shifting her remarks to her present husband, neither preceding nor following this ploy by details that would elaborate or locate this sudden shift. Nothing was said about how long the husband had experienced periodic impotence nor about the significance the woman attached to the situation. There is no simple way to code the response unless we first provide an elaboration that claims to locate the remarks in a larger context of past relationships with the husband. Do we view the remark as an attempt to help the interviewer "understand" the wife's predicament with her husband, or to give some kind of answer to a question the respondent did not understand or was trying to avoid? We could construct many possible interpretations to locate this "answer." We might imply that because the information is "intimate," the interviewer has been "successful" in establishing "rapport" with the respondent. Or, we might simply assume that the sudden shift to present sexual problems means that the woman had to tell (or had been hoping to tell) somebody about her situation. One possible way of clarifying this dilemma is to search for other "evidence" in the interview that might support one of our interpretations; but the search would again require us to modify our questionnaire format in which questions (stimuli) motivate answers (responses) in an orderly way.

All the questions on premarital relationships were designed to induce the respondent to reveal information about himself or herself that a fixed-choice question either would preclude or would structure in such a way that the respondent could choose an "appropriate" answer without indicating to the researcher whether the respondent had given any thought to the issue before it came up during the interview.

Consider the following questions, which were designed to elicit from the elderly respondent further details about the premarital activities that had led to her marriage.

The questioning began by asking whether the respondent and her present spouse had discussed marriage during their courtship.

4. INTERVIEWER. Did you (the two of you) ever talk about getting married? (FA 7 MU 1-21;g) [At some time did (the two) of you talk about getting married?]
   RESPONDENT. Yes.

The brief answer "yes" tells us almost nothing. A fixed-choice answer of "seldom," "occasionally," or "often" would have told us very little more. We cannot reconstruct the behavioral scenes that may or may not have occurred and are now subsumed under the response "yes."

Probe   What did you say?
5. RESPONDENT. That if he had good intention (s) I would accept him. I was distrustful (of him) because there are men with bad intentions. "If you come with good intentions I accept, if not, no." [As if she were telling the interviewer how she spoke to her husband to be.] I treated him with *Usted* [formally—by using the polite form of address]. I treated him this way [formally] for 2 or 3 months. After 2 or 3 months when we became "promised" to each other (engaged to be married), we began to *tutear*. [We became intimate on a first-name basis, using the familiar form of address.]

The probe asked what the woman would or did say at the time. Her reply to the probe suggests a "proper" relationship whereby the man was presumably told he would be accepted if he had good intentions. The respondent's comments can be viewed as an attempt to reconstruct the treatment accorded to the husband-to-be. She provides commonsense evidence of a "proper" relationship by reference to her insistence on polite forms of address until two or three months had passed and the couple were engaged to be married. But we have no other details about their day-to-day physical and verbal communication. The age of the couple may have been one reason for the seemingly exaggerated formality of the relationship, or perhaps the woman was simply afraid of men, as suggested earlier; perhaps, too, all courtships were more formal at the time the couple met. Or, there may have been a combination of these three or even a dozen more possibilities. The particular statements we call questions and answers are sufficiently ambiguous, yet they also seem sufficiently plausible to allow us to construct a rather large number of "convincing" explanations.

The question–answer format is convenient and is considered to be an acceptable way of communicating information in an ordered way. The central point is that the question–answer format *creates* misleading "appropriate" outcomes. The format is a practical and self-organizing common sense or members' procedure which can be extended indefinitely to provide for arbitrary cutoff points that can be justified as "enough," "too much," and so on.

Let me illustrate this members' procedure by referring to the questions on courtship, picking out features of the previous dialogue that depict a convincing historical account.

6. INTERVIEWER. How did you come to marry him? (FA 7 MU 1-21;h)
   RESPONDENT. [They became married at the outset. The interviewer did not write down the answer verbatim, but paraphrased the respondent's remarks.]

The question asking how the woman came to marry her husband did not produce a "clear" answer, but the interviewer seemed to paraphrase an "answer" by stating that they were married "at the outset." The question was ambiguous, and the interviewer was negligent in failing to write down a verbatim response—or perhaps the respondent tried to avoid an answer. The next question was:

7. INTERVIEWER. What made you want to be married to him (FA 7 MU 1-21;i)
   RESPONDENT. Because I worked, and it is very difficult to stay employed;

> it is better to work in one's own home. I would have liked to
> marry a man but the opportunity never presented itself.

This question seemed to force the respondent into a more direct reply.
The earlier question was a standard one, asked throughout the questionnaire, and designed to encourage a kind of free association whereby
spontaneous details about the marriage might be elicited. We could say
that the strategy failed here; thus the next question was intended to force
the issue to provide "evidence" that could be used in the analysis. The
respondent's answer seemed to be quite practical, hence "convincing."
She stated she worked and that it was difficult to stay employed, and
that it was 'better to work in one's own home.' She went on to say that
she would have liked to have married a man earlier, but that the opportunity never presented itself.

8. *Probe.*   Surely you did not help them (men) find you, were you
afraid of them?
RESPONDENT.   Yes, I was afraid of them.
Probe.   Why were you afraid of them?
RESPONDENT.   Because of what people would say. In addition my mother
would always tell me to be careful because men always want
to fool (trick) one. [Men always try and deceive girls (or
trick them) into having sexual relations with them.]

Here the interviewer appeared to be dissatisfied with the previous answer
and pushed the respondent by asking her if she had tried to block efforts
on the part of men to meet her, and if she was afraid of men. The woman
said she was afraid of men because of what 'people' said about them,
and that her mother told her to be careful because '. . . men always want
to fool (trick) one.'

The interviewer *did not* (and probably never would have) asked the
woman if she "were getting old and afraid that she might never land a
man, so she finally grabbed this one for convenience." The question–
answer format only tacitly presumes that the unstated conditions of the
setting and the way in which the participants develop a sense of the
"permissible" will dictate how far the interviewer can deviate from
"polite" questions and answers. For example:

9. INTERVIEWER.   Did the marriage have something to do with your being
pregnant? (FA 7 MU 1-21;l)
RESPONDENT.   I did not have (sexual) relations before getting married.

INTERVIEWER. Who was more interested (anxious) in getting married? (FA 7 MU 1-21;m)

RESPONDENT. He was more interested because his daughter was leaving home, because she was getting married and only he and his sons would remain at home.

The questions about the possibility of a pregnancy having hastened the marriage, and about who was more interested in getting married seem to provide additional "convincing" material that the union was a practical one for both partners. The woman shifted from her practical circumstances to the husband's, implying that with the married daughter gone, there would not be a woman around to take care of the men. The formal interview questions could never reveal the variety of possible interpretations that we might regard as convincing. I think it would be useful to pursue the issue by describing further remarks made by the same woman about her marriage.

The wife had listened to various parts of the husband's interview and had learned for the first time that he had had three steady girlfriends before he met her; and this annoyed her so much that she told the interviewer she would give similar details about her life. The wife revealed that her distrust of men stemmed from having had to work hard as a servant and cook after the death of her father. She had met many other servants who had told her stories about women being abandoned by men after the women became pregnant. The interviewer seemed quite convinced when the woman recounted such "intimate" episodes. The interviewer was particularly impressed when the woman contradicted the husband's claim that he had not used contraceptives. The respondent said the husband had not wanted any more children and had used contraceptives, whereas she had wanted at least one child.

I have not releated with direct quotations the lengthy account given by the interviewer of what was undoubtedly an even longer account by the respondent. I assume, as the interviewer did, that the woman was really "opening up," providing details about the couple's sexual life, about her frustrations, the husband's impotence, her fears of men; yet very few particulars are reproduced here. If the lengthy particulars available were presented, some readers would complain that too much detail was given, and others might say that such details were "rich" and convincing. I have tried to argue that whereas some details are relevant for some readers, many readers would prefer a tabulated account representing large numbers of respondents but ignoring the inherent ambiguity and misleading "hardness" of data coded from material from fixed-choice and open-ended questions. Other readers would be content to read about a few cases in which "rich" details are provided. Neither type of reader may be satisfied with the observation that "rich" particulars and tabulated accounts overlook the possibility for tacit cooperation between interviewer and respondent in producing accounts that seem "reasonable" for the practical purpose of getting through the interview and writing a convincing report.

How the Setting Reformulates Planned Questionnaire Discourse. The next case, taken at random, is of interest because of the way in which the woman seems to have convinced the interviewer that the information elicited is the "truth," even though her husband might say something different. The woman respondent explained the discrepancy in their answers with *"Ud. sabe como son los hombres"*—"You know how men are. . . ." The interviewers's feelings about the relationship established were central in the making of decisions throughout the interview about whether to probe further, whether further probing would be dangerous, whether the question had been answered "satisfactorily," and whether the respondent was "lying" or telling the "truth."

In this case the interviewer began to make judgments during the interview about the success and credibility of the interview. The interview was spread out over several occasions and required eight hours to complete. The family lived in a working-class suburb, and the round trip from downtown Buenos Aires required the interviewer to travel about three hours. At first the husband refused to be interviewed by the interviewer. I then spent almost two months trying to see him to discuss the matter. I finally succeeded in reaching the husband and we spoke for almost two hours, but he still declined to be interviewed, saying that it was of no interest to him and that he was too busy. When I learned that the man was the director of a union local in the city, I tried to study the local and some of the families from the factory, thus becoming quite friendly with him. I learned a great deal about the husband during informal conversations, but I could not ask questions and record answers formally during an interview.

All the interaction incidents described below included the interviewer's assessment of whether the party was "sincere," "truthful," "lying," "naïve," "comprehending," and the like, and these judgments influenced the manner in which questions were asked and answers were formulated as the scene unfolded. The assessments occurred throughout the interview. Although interviewer and respondent develop initial orientations, these can be altered at any time as "new" evidence is received or "old" evidence is linked retrospectively to present particulars (or vice versa). The interviewer may probe more, may suspect the relevance of certain particulars, or may feel that the respondent is "really opening up." The respondent may be especially careful in producing accounts (answers) at different junctures throughout the interview.

The interviewer's account of her encounter with the wife proceeded as follows:

10. I rang the bell three times. A woman answered from behind a "peekhole" (an opening in the door, about 3 × 5 inches) covered with a wire screen woven very compactly. I saw absolutely nothing. This [situation] gave the impression of talking with a monastic nun. I had to make an effort to smile because it was like smiling at the wall. It turned out to be the woman of the house. She asked several times what it [the interview] was for, telling me that she was about to go out. I told her I could come back whenever she would say to. She said to come back at any time. I asked her to please concretize the time. She asked once again what it [the interview] was for. I asked her to let me show her the papers. She said: "One moment, I'll be back." She returned in a short time and she had me enter [the house]. I had to dodge a lighted heater that was just next to the door. As soon as the door was closed, [the respondent] the lady of the house turned out to be friendly. She tried to explain to me how does one know whether one should answer? [the questions] I clarified for her that we were interested in what she thought about certain things. Her son came, a young man of some 14, 15 years, of whom I asked if he was already enrolled in the university (trying to obtain his sympathy, since he appeared to be the "star" of the house, and including the one whom the mother saw as an authority in these matters). I left it that I would return on Tuesday the 29th of October for her and one day in the morning for the husband. We'll see what happens.

The interviewer implied that the opening exchange was difficult because of the wire screen portion of the door through which she was forced to address the respondent. I presume that the respondent's suggestion that the interviewer "come back at any time" could be taken as a means of putting off the interviewer. I also presume that the interviewer's request that the woman specify a time for an interview was an attempt to avoid endless visits and also to investigate the possibility of a reject. We could claim that offering to show credentials was "comforting" to the respondent, but it would be just as easy to claim that information not expressed verbally was more convincing to the respondent, who may have been positively swayed by the interviewer's appearance and "friendly" manner.

The interviewer's observation that the first brief interview "turned out to be friendly," coupled with her remarks that the respondent was perhaps concerned about whether "she could answer" appropriately, sound plausible. We can interpret the interviewer's remarks to imply that she was let into the house so that the son could check her out and perhaps assure the mother. Apparently the interviewer was only partly optimistic about the possible success of the interview, though there are few "convincing" details since her statement "We'll see what happens" seems to suggest doubts about ever completing the interview.

11. TUESDAY. I ring the bell several times; in a short time a neighbor appears who tells me that the woman's mother became ill, that she does not know when she will return, that the husband will come to sleep [at the house]. I tell her that I will return and she asks me, 'And if she does not come back for a month?' (I smell a reject, I don't know, we shall see.)

THURSDAY, November 7. We arrived with Professor Cicourel in the morning, we surprised her half asleep. She told me I should return in the afternoon (and) that she would attend me (grant me the interview). That she had to go out, but that she would wait for me (later).

THURSDAY AFTERNOON. At last. She let me enter and it turned out the reverse of what I had thought (expected). Altogether warm, continually asking that she be forgiven (excused) because of not having attended (granted an interview to) me before. The first part of the interview was done at a high price. She would ask, What is it for? Especially on the questions about salary. After telling the answer she said to me: "Look I tell you the truth. My husband may very well tell you differently but you know how men are. . . ." (FA 10 MU-10)

In the foregoing report, we can see how certain particulars were used by the interviewer to communicate a possible "reject" and how the interviewer then reversed her view to "feel" that the respondent was quite "truthful" about her responses. The interviewer's account of the respondent's answers combines the former's thoughts written before, during, and after the interview, but it does not reveal how questions and answers were influenced by each party's conception of the exchange, at each moment. Nor can we speak of the "real reasons" behind a question (or behind the entire interview) or of the "truthfulness" of a particular answer.

Doubts experienced during the initial attempts to obtain entrance, as well as doubts that may arise during the interview, may be linked retrospectively to decisions about how to manage some portions of the questionnaire. The doubts may lead the interviewer not to ask certain probes or to decide that certain matters require probes. It is very difficult to record interviewer doubts as they unfold, connecting them with the interviewer's changing perceptions of the credibility of the responses offered. It is even more difficult to infer the respondent's doubts about what the "real" intentions of the interview are, or her doubts about the meaning or possible negative consequences of answering specific questions in certain ways.

The accounts produced by the question–answer format can be analyzed in several ways. Our procedure is to demonstrate how moment-to-moment contingencies of the setting, as articulated with the memory of past events, produce the accounts we label "data," whereas traditional methodology treats the questions and answers as context-free displays of abstract social structures.

Turning to the scheduled questions, the interviewer asked the woman about premarital relations and sexual unions, and we find the following exchange.

12. INTERVIEWER. How many young men did you go with? (FA 10 MU 10;19a)
    RESPONDENT. Only my husband because I had a *filito* when I was 15 years old; kid stuff. [The translation of *filito* is difficult, but it refers to a minor "affair" that does not involve sexual relations.]

The questioning began with the interviewer asking about the number of young men the respondent had been courted by. Her reply ("kid stuff") is of interest because it initially characterized her premarital experience as being virtually nil.

13. INTERVIEWER. Do you remember anything about the first young man with whom you went out? (FA 10 MU-10;19c)
    RESPONDENT. I was 15 years old, more or less.
    INTERVIEWER. What was it that you liked about him? (19d)
    RESPONDENT. The character (personality) he had. A very refined young man, very delicate (frail?). All (everything) different from my husband.
    INTERVIEWER. How old were you when you began to go out with him? (19e)
    RESPONDENT. 15 years.
    INTERVIEWER. Did he work? At what? (19f)

RESPONDENT. He was a musician of the army barracks. He was a corporal. He was a military man.

INTERVIEWER. Did you work? (19g)

RESPONDENT. No.

INTERVIEWER. Did your family know that you were going out with him? (19h)

RESPONDENT. No. It was done (the going out) very little.

INTERVIEWER. How would your family feel about this relationship if they had known about it? (19i)

RESPONDENT. They would have liked him. The only one who found out after a year was my aunt. They would have liked him because he was a very good (nice) young man, from a good family.

14. INTERVIEWER. Did they talk to you about the young man? (19j)

RESPONDENT. No, because they found out after (later, it was over).

INTERVIEWER. What did they say to you? (19k)

RESPONDENT. My little sister liked him (it).

Her recollection of the young musician could be taken to be a kind of romantic exaggeration. The interviewer suggested to me that the respondent was using the episode to suggest her unhappiness with her husband. The respondent seemed to be preoccupied with giving the interviewer a highly favorable impression of the young man ("a very refined young man"; "they (the family) would have liked him because he was a very good (nice) young man, from a good family"). There is no discussion of how the young man's family was judged to be "good," nor are there additional details about the husband's family. New particulars easily alter the significance of prior particulars. No convincing interpretation is possible here, but we could say, following the interviewer's suggestion, that the respondent was currently unhappy with her husband and thus exaggerated the account to the interviewer of the early courtship incident. This theme seems to become more convincing below. The interviewer's retrospective report of the woman's relationship with her husband provided me with an ad hoc basis for interpreting the interview material.

15. INTERVIEWER. Did your mother know that you were going out with this young man? (19l)

RESPONDENT. No. [She wasn't living with her mother at this time.]

INTERVIEWER. What would she have thought if she had known about it? (19m)

RESPONDENT. She would have liked him (it).

One line of questioning is doggedly pursued by the interviewer in trying to elicit information about the parental reaction to the boyfriend. The questionnaire continues as follows:

16. INTERVIEWER. (If the mother did not know about the existence of the young man, ask:) Why didn't your mother know that you were going out with him? (Regardless of the question, keep on asking:) Could you tell me more about this? (19p)

RESPONDENT. I was living with my grandmother and my grandfather. Heaven forbid that I say something about it!

INTERVIEWER. Where and with whom did you live before beginning to go out with him? (19q)

RESPONDENT. With my grandparents. I think that he would have been the man for me. I am happy with my husband now because I adjusted (adapted) myself. But I cried (so) a lot. He [her husband, I presume] is not like me. At times he is nice (well) and suddenly he becomes mean (bad). The other one (musician) was such a refined young man. At times I regret having married so young. If only I had been able to go out (dating) even for two years. My husband married when he was almost 30, he was already tired of living. I had not started (to live). (In the questions about courtship, she says that I will have to write a lot about her husband. She says that she is going to spy [on our interviewing]. She also says that she knows that he went with a gal as a girlfriend [who was like a girlfriend or sweetheart]).

The questions permitted the respondent to elaborate an answer in a way that revealed that she had been raised by her grandparents. We might treat her references to the grandparents as a way of telling the interviewer that they were so strict, that questions about premarital sexual relations were irrelevant. Or, we could have been told by the interviewer that the woman "seemed" to be the "type" who could have been "promiscuous," whereupon we might assume that through subtle glances and intonation the respondent sensed this and kept implying a home atmosphere of strictness on the part of the grandparents as a means of "answering" these "invisible" charges.

When the respondent was asked "Where and with whom did you live before beginning to go out with him?" she answered "With my grandparents." But added, apropos of nothing contained in the stimulus question, "I think that he would have been the man for me. I am happy with my husband now because I adjusted (adapted) myself. But I cried (so) a lot." It is not clear which "man" she meant. She seemed to refer to the boyfriend as "the man for me," then commenting with apparent resignation on her present marriage. Her remarks can be construed as disparaging to her husband, although they seem to justify her present marriage.

18. INTERVIEWER. How often did you see each other? Where? (19w)

RESPONDENT. Not even for two minutes at the door because I couldn't because I was with my grandparents. I was brought up well (strictly) so that I did not have the nerve to be seen with him during errands. No. May God help me. My grandfather was very severe (strict). I was quite afraid of my grandfather.

INTERVIEWER. Did you ever have sexual relations with him? [the young man] (19x)

RESPONDENT. No.

[Here she remarks that at the moment of the questions, she at times does not know how to answer, but that later she remembers and for example says:] When you asked me If I would like to live with the children (when I am old) —I would like to live with the children. When you asked me this [I didn't ask it of her] I told you no. (For my part) I would like to live with them. I get along with them so well, I dance, I am like a crazy person. But of course I think about their wives. [*She is already jealous in anticipation.*] My husband likes to dance and he does it quite well. He dances a lot with a sister-in-law and everyone watches them. I don't dance with him because—[I don't know how?] I don't know, why should everyone look at me and see that I do it poorly, right?

My husband provides us with everything we need, but he is not a companion to the children. I see this neighbor that talks to them [talks to his own children? or the respondent's?] He never does. I have to talk to my children. For example, I question the eldest. He says to me "Mother, I don't like you asking me these things." But if I don't do it who will? I asked him the other day if he had ever kissed a girl and he told me (that he had) twice here and here (on the forehead and on the cheek).

Do these answers mean that the respondent "trusts" the interviewer? Do they signify a deep unhappiness with the marriage? Are these remarks a "sign" of neurotic marital adjustment? Are the wife's fairly detailed complaints attributable to a recent argument between the husband and wife—that is, if the interview had happened to fall a month earlier or later, would the responses have been different?

If we treat the questions and answers as "objective" manifestations of real experiences that are independent of our research methods for eliciting them, and independent of both the situated interaction and the relationship between respondent and interviewer, we will encounter a few difficulties producing tables summarizing our data (number of premarital unions, e.g.). To admit that there are contextual particulars and that these particulars are presupposed by the ways in which talk is socially organized, by nonverbal features of the setting, or by the way in which answers are generated by selective attention and memory, is to invite structural chaos into traditional analysis.

We could readily claim that the respondent's remarks about her husband suggest considerable ambivalence about her marriage and about the husband's relationship with her and the children. ("At times I regret having married so young. If only I had been able to go out (dating) even for two years. My husband married when he was almost 30, he was already tired of living. I had not started (to live).") We cannot clearly know the chronological history of these doubts relative to their inner-time reconstruction. We might speculate that the interview provided the occasion for reviewing the respondent's entire life or, alternatively, that such negative remarks about the husband revealed only recent conflicts. We could claim that because such detailed questions may be seldom discussed by respondents during day-to-day living, our questions motivate the remarks said to be of substantive interest. (Compare the case of a patient who goes to a therapist to *discover* the specific problems that presumably justify the therapy.)

Interviews like the one just presented could suggest how unlikely premarital relations were at the time of the respondent's youth, or that some marriages were a way to escape from difficult family conditions. Such an interview could also suggest that occasions for reviewing a marriage can produce variable reconstructions, but the sources of this variability are not accessible to the researcher by a strict question–answer format. At the time a question is asked, the respondent may not be able to process the information or may not want to formulate an answer; later in the exchange, however, she may feel that she can trust the interviewer, or that she now understands one or more possible intentions of the question.

Conclusions. The second interviewer's remarks indicate why she first doubted, then she believed, that it would be possible to have the interview. These remarks also suggest the basis for the credence placed in the informant. Note how the interviewer's doubts emerged during the first encounter, how she returned to find a neighbor hinting that an interview might never materialize ("I smell a reject, I don't know, we shall see.") but on the third day (and fourth visit) it all turned out "different." The interviewer also reported that the wife said that the husband's responses were not necessarily to be believed. The interviewer supplies various particulars to compose a convincing account. This means that as readers we will look for and organize particulars we think index broader aspects of meaning to find a believable conclusion. I do something similar when I call the reader's attention to specific points mentioned by the interviewer and elaborate on them to guide the reader through my construction of what happened. The language used by the interviewer incorporates particulars used by her and by the respondent during the initial exchanges. I, in turn, make use of some of these particulars in my elaboration of the interviewer's account.

I have sought to show how the moment-to-moment perceptions and decision-making of both interviewer and respondent generate an environment of objects that is self-organizing. The interviewer's questions and the respondent's answers furnish materials for making this environment of socially defined objects a reified normative reconstruction. The respondent finds her problems in the questions, even though the questions are often merely vehicles for pushing her into reviewing her past and present (and possibly future) practical circumstances. If the questions remain open ended, they also serve the researcher in his search for intentions and experiences that can reformulate the problem selectively but cannot be asked about directly. If the questions provide only fixed-choice responses, both the researcher's and the respondent's tasks are easier, yet misleading.

To understand possible meanings of family organization and fertility behavior in an everyday context, we must recognize that it is through reflexive talk and nonverbal information that we simultaneously produce and discover the everyday world as members and as member-researchers.

APPENDIX.   SPANISH VERSION OF INTERVIEW MATERIALS

1. Q: ¿Qué hacía?
   A: Lo recibia en mi casa, él venía a la nochecita dos (?) veces por semana. Mis padres eran muy delicados. (FA 7 MUI-19;o)

2. Q: ¿ Con qué frecuencia se veían? ¿Dónde?

   A: Cada 15 dias o 20 porque los padres eran 'delicados,' no querían que se vieran todos los días." (FA 7 MU1-19;w)

3. Q: ¿Podría decirme algo más acerca de esto?

   A: Mi actual marido quiere tener relaciones cada 4 días, pero no puede y se pone muy nervioso. Lo intenta cuando está bien pero no cuando está enojado. Entonces se da vuelta para la pared. (FA 7 MU1-19;y)

4. Q: ¿Hablaban Uds. alguna vez de casarse? (FA 7 MU1; 21g)

   A: Si.

5. *Probe.* ¿Qué decía Ud?

   A: Que si tenía buena intención lo aceptaría. Yo desconfiaba, porque hay hombres con malas intenciones. "Si Ud. viene con buenos intenciones lo accepto, si no, no." [As if she were telling the interviewer how she spoke to her husband to be.] Yo lo trataba de Ud. Así lo traté 2 o 3 meses. Cuando nos comprometimos después de 2 o 3 meses, empezamos a tutearnos.

6. Q: ¿Cómo llegó a casarse con él? (21;h)

   A: [Se casaron al comienzo.] (The interviewer did not write down the answer verbatim, but paraphrased the respondent's remarks.)

7. Q: ¿Qué le hacía querer casarse con él? (21;i)

   A: Porque yo trabajaba, y es muy pesado estar empleada; mejor trabajar en la casa de uno. Me hubiera gustado casarme con un hombre pero no se presentó la opportunidad.

8. *Probe.* ¿Seguramente Ud. no les ayudaba a encontrarla, les tendría miedo?

   A: Si, les tenía miedo.

   Probe. ¿Porqué les tenía miedo?

   A: Por lo que la gente decía. Ademés mi madre siempre me decía ·que me cuidará porque los hombres siempre la quieren engañar a una.

9. Q: ¿Tuvo algo que ver quedar (dejarla) embarazada con el casamiento? (21;l)

   A: No tuvo relaciones antes de casarme.

   Q: ¿Quién estaba más intersado en casarse? (21;m)

   A: Él tenía más interés porque se le iba la hija de su casa, porque se casaba y en la casa solo quedaban él y sus hijos varones.

10. Toqué el timbre tres veces. Respondío a través de una murilla

cubierta con un alambre tejido muy tupido, una mujer. Yo no veía absolutamente nada. Daba la impresión de estar hablando con una monja de clausura. Me tuve que esforzar para sonreir, porque era como sonreirle a la pared. Resultó ser la Sra. de la casa. Preguntó para que era varias veces, diciéndome que estaba por salir. Le dije que volviera en cualquier momento. Le pedí por favor que me concretarà el momento. Otra vez preguntó para que era. Le pedí que me permitiera mostrarle la credencial. Me dijo: 'Un momento, ya vuelvo.' Volvío al ratito y me hizo pasar. Tuve que sortear estufa prendida que estaba justo junto a la puerta. Una vez franqueada la puerta la Sra. resultó amable. Trataba de explicarme ¿que cómo uno sabe si sabría contestar? Le aclaré que nos interesaba lo que ella pensaba sobre ciertas cosas. Vino el hijo, un jovencito de unos 14, 15 años al que pregunté si ya estaba en la Universidad (tratando de lograr su simpatía, puesto que parecía el ilustrado de la casa, e incluso hacia quien la madre vera como autoridad en estas cosas). Quedé en volver el martes 29 de octubre, para ella y algun día a la mañana para el esposo. Veremos que pasa.

11. MARTES. Tocó el timbre varias veces, al rato aparece una vecina que me dice que a la Sra. se le enfermó la mamá, que no sabe cuando volverá, que el marido vendrá a dormir. Le digo que voy a volver y me pregunta. "¿Y si tarda un mes?' 'Me huele a rechazo, no sé, veremos).

JUEVES 7 DE NOVIEMBRE. Llegamos con el Prof. Cicourel a la mañana, la sorprendimos media dormida. Me dijo que volviera a la tarde que me iba atender. Que tenía que salir, pero que me iba a esperar.

JUEVES A LA TARDE. Al fin. Me hizo pasar y resultó al revés de lo que yo pensaba. Sumamente calida, pidiendo permanentemente disculpas (disimuladamente) de no haberme atendido antes. Costó mucho la primera parte de la entrevista. ¿Preguntaba para que es? Sobre todo en las preguntas de sueldo. Después de decirlo me dijo: Mire yo le digo la verdad. Mi esposo a lo mejor le dice distinto pero Ud. sabe como son los hombres . . ." (FA 10 MU-10)

12. Q: ¿Con cuántos muchachos anduvo Ud? (FA 10-MU 10;19a)
    A: Mi marido solamente porque tuve un filito cuando tenía 15 años; cosas de chicos.

13. Q: ¿Ud. se acuerda del primer muchacho con el que anduvo? (19c)
    A: Más o menos, tenía 15 años.

Q: ¿Qué le gustaba en él? (19d)

A: El caracter. Un muchacho muy fino, muy delicado. Todo lo distinto de mi marido.

Q: Qué edad tenía Ud. cuando comenzó a andar con él? (19e)

A: 15 años.

Q: ¿El trabajaba? ¿en qué? (19f)

A: Era músico del cuartel. Era cabo. Era militar.

Q: ¿Ud. trabajaba (19g)

A: No.

Q: ¿Sabía su familia que Ud. andaba con él? (19h)

A: No. Fue poquito.

Q: ¿Qué opinión tenía su familia sobre esa relación (o hubiera tenido) si hubiera sabido acerca de ella? (19i)

A: Y se le hubiese gustado. La única que se enteró al año fue mi tía. Les hubiera gustado porque era un muchacho muy bien, de buena familia.

14. Q: ¿Le hablaban sobre el muchacho? (19j)

A: No, porque se enteraron después.

Q: ¿Qué le decían? (19k)

A: Ami hermanita le gustaba.

15. Q: ¿Sabía su madre que Ud. andaba con ese muchacho? (19l)

A: No. [Ella no vivía con la madre en ese momento.]

Q: ¿Qué pensaba (qué hubiera pensado si lo hubiera sabido)? (19m)

A: Le hubiese gustado.

16. Q: (Si la madre no sabía de la existencia del muchacho, preguntar:) ¿Por qué no sabía su madre que Ud. andaba con él? (Sea, cual fuera la pregunta, insista preguntando:) ¿Podría decirme algo más? (19p)

A: Yo estaba con mi abuelita y mi abuelo. ¿Dios me libre de decírselo?

Q: ¿Dónde y con quién vivía Ud. antes de comenzar a salir con él? (19q)

A: Con los abuelos. Yo creo que el hubiera sido el hombre para mí. Yo soy feliz, con mi esposo ahora porque me amolde. Pero lloré tanto. Él no es como yo. A veces está bien y de pronto se pon mal. Él otro era muchacho tan fino. A veces me arrepiento de haberme casado tan joven. Si hubiera podido salir aunque fuera 2 años. Mi esposo cuando se casó tenía casi 30 años, ya estaba cansado de vivir. Yo no había empezado. [En las preguntas de noviazgos, dice que para el marido va a haber que escribir tanto. Dice que ella va a espiar. Dice también que ella sabe que anduvo con una chica de novio.]

17. Q: ¿Vivío alguna vez con él? (19r)

A: No.

Q: ¿Por que no vivío con él?

A: Fue muy poco tiempo. Era muy chica. Huy! si le pregunta a mi marido. (Dice que cuando le pregunten al marido ella va a espiar. Me parece que está un poco orgullosa de la experiencia amorosa de su esposo y un poco envidiosa.)

Q: ¿Alguna vez pensó en vivir con él? (Indagar) (¿Podría decirme algo más acerca de esto?) (19u)

A: No. ¿Sabe cuàndo yo me avivé? A mi me avivó mi marido. ¿Era una caída del catre?

Q: ¿Habló alguna vez de matrimonio con él? (19v)

A: No. Si ni hablaba siquiera.

18. Q: ¿Con qué frecuencia se veían? ¿Dónde? (19w)

A: Ni dos minutos en la puerta porque no podía porque estaba con abuelos. Estaba bien criada así que no tenía la picardia de verme con él en los mandados. No. Dios me libre. Mi abuelo era muy severo. Yo le tenía mucho miedo a mi abuelo.

Q: ¿Tuvo alguna vez relaciones sexuales con él? (19x)

A: No.

[Acá comenta que en el momento de las preguntas a veces no sabe que contestar, pero que luego se acuerda y dice por ejemplo.] "Cuando Ud. me preguntó si me gustaría vivir con los chicos." Me gustaría vivir con los chicos. Cuando Ud. me preguntó eso (Yo no se lo pregunté) yo le dije que no. A mi me gustaría vivir con ellos. Me llevo tan bien, bailo, me hago la loca. Pero claro pienso en las esposas. [Ya está celosa por anticipado.] A mi marido le gusta bailar y lo hace muy bien. Baila mucho con una cuñada y, todas los miran. ¿yo no bailo con él porque no sé, para qué los demás me miren y ven que lo hago mal, no?

Mi esposo no nos hace falta nada, pero no es compañero de los hijos. Yo veo ese vecino que les habla. El nunca. Yo les tengo que hablar a mis hijos. Por ejemplo al mayor yo le pregunto. Él me dice, "Mamá no me gusta que me preguntes esas cosas," ¿pero si no quién le va a hablar? Le pregunté el otra día si había besado a alguna chica y me dijo que dos veces acá y acá [en la frente y en la mejilla].

CHAPTER 7

CONTRASTING PERSPECTIVES
IN THE ANALYSIS OF MATERIALS

In this chapter I present a series of tables assembled from the interview materials in my study of Argentine fertility. The tables indicate resources we can use for gathering evidence to support certain traditional arguments (e.g., that the desire for small families, as expressed in the questionnaire responses, is evidenced by the small size of actual families). I have tabulated the answers from the open-ended questions to show the limitations of the survey approach.

I contrast inferences made possible by coding the open-ended responses with those obtained by an indirect textual analysis of the same responses. Both types of inferences require the researcher to refer to the contingencies of the interaction which are necessary for obtaining, bounding, and eliciting information. The interactional particulars that produce the interview materials can only be described in a selective way because most of the interviews were recorded by hand, and even the transcripts of tape-recorded sessions do not convey the subtleties of the nonverbal communication. Our understanding of the audio tapes of the "original" scene is constrained by a vocabulary and a syntax that are presumed to be invariant vis-á-vis the perspective from which the recording equipment is operated. The researcher's descriptions of the interviews, and the respondent's descriptions of the "original" scenes, introduce selective elements into our account of the events.

The researcher's use of the particulars he selectively labels "data" is part of a broader activity whereby he sustains an everyday existence within which the research proceeds and on which he trades implicitly. Every description of scientific activity relies on this existence, even though the researcher does not acknowledge that he must sustain this commonsense world in connection with his claims to knowledge about an environment of objects that relies on implicit, culturally organized verbal and nonverbal conditions. The discussion of the tables and interview materials that follows seeks to incorporate the researcher's reliance on his commonsense knowledge and reasoning into the description of the findings.

In Chapter 6 I used Table 1 (p. 92) to illustrate how information is lost in moving from the original questions and answers to traditional tables that are presumed to be concise summaries of research findings. The results of that table might suggest, for example that fertility is restricted because of the length of courtship, particularly if there is little premarital intercourse and if there are attempts to prevent pregnancy.

Although I have described some of the substantive conclusions about sexual unions that can be inferred from the interview materials, I have not suggested that Argentine courtship appears to be somewhat longer than North American courtship, or that the Table mentioned will be misleading unless the entries are recorded to reveal length of courtship periods that ended in marriage and the respondents' age at marriage. Traditional analysis would suggest that we should be able to relate existing economic conditions to length of courship and age at marriage.

Traditional sociological researchers refer to length of courtship (Table 1, Chapter 6) as a dependent variable that is associated with such independent variables as (a) the financial conditions of the couple, (b) their need to terminate courtship because of pregnancy, (c) their ability to abstain from sexual relations or to engage in them with the use of contraceptives (perhaps holding "constant" variables like ignorance of such use and/or religious beliefs), (d) the role of fortuitous elements (e.g., an occasion leading to the decision to elope or to shorten plans made with the parents), or (e) the motivation of one party to have an early marriage because of a desire to have sexual relations or to be assured that there is more to courtship than talk about love.

Contrasting Views of Traditional Data. Demographers begin their discussion of fertility by referring to the activity of sexual contact based on cohabitation, the respondents' physiological obstacles to childbirth or conception, and economic difficulties and belief system constraints that result in differential motivation to produce children. By asking questions about family size, the researcher presumes that married couples routinely give thought to the number of children desired. A corollary of the presumption that couples are concerned with family size is the idea that married persons will have intelligent reason either for desiring a specific number of children or for being content to accept "all that God sends." Correlational studies require research procedures that preclude or eliminate meanings for the respondent that are inherently vague or multiple. Thus situated meanings cannot be conceived, much less coded. The idea that a good "feeling" toward the interviewer or toward the last "answer" may be the basis for the next response does not sit well if we assume that each question (presented in a randomized way) is designed to tap existing conceptions neatly stored in the subject's belief or knowledge system.

As a rule, the researcher's pretest questions about family size are open-ended. When researchers ask fixed-choice questions, they assume that most of the responses the subjects are likely to give have been presented and that an "other" category will subsume the few respondents with more unusual replies. The survey questionnaire includes stimulus sentences that can be identified easily by the respondent as meaningful, but it also allows the researcher to cross-tabulate items that, presumably, are not linked together by the respondent. If when we ask for the respondent's ideal family size we have also recorded the number of children conceived, we can reason that any discrepancy in the two numbers is of theoretical and practical interest. The theoretical interest emerges from a concern with reproduction motives and beliefs, and practical reforms or programs become possible if means can be found for assisting those who desire small families. If actual family size is small but motives are revealed that suggest the couple would like a larger family, we can reason that belief considerations are secondary to other considerations, such as economic difficulties in the family.

Considering Table 1, we could say that except for women with secondary education (a small part of our sample), the major part of the respondents desired small families. In compiling Table 1, ideal family size was indexed by asking the respondent

What size family do you think is best?
¿Cuál cree Ud. qué es el mejor tamaño de una familia?

It appears obvious in Table 1 that more men and women in our sample preferred three or fewer children than preferred four or more. But the table is rather cumbersome to read and the table entries too small for us to say more about ideal family size. By conveniently combining categories, we can produce Table 1A and perhaps convince the reader that men and women with little education seem to prefer as few children as men with

TABLE 1. IDEAL FAMILY SIZE BY AGE AND EDUCATION

Number of Respondents in Each Age/Education Category

Ideal Family Size	No Education 30 or less	No Education Over 30	Primary Incomplete 30 or less	Primary Incomplete Over 30	Primary Completed 30 or less	Primary Completed Over 30	Secondary Incomplete 30 or less	Secondary Incomplete Over 30	Secondary Completed 30 or less	Secondary Completed Over 30	University Incomplete 30 or less	University Incomplete Over 30	University Completed 30 or less	University Completed Over 30	Totals
Men[a]															
3 children or fewer	—	2	3	24	3	14	2	7	—	4	—	2	—	8	69
4 or more children	—	1	—	11	1	7	1	1	—	1	—	—	—	7	30
															99
Women[b]															
3 children or fewer	—	3	6	31	9	27	2	4	4	7	1	1	—	2	97
4 or more children	—	3	2	18	2	11	1	5	2	7	—	1	—	—	52
															149

[a] 7 cases stated they wanted 3–4 children and these were coded as 3; 1 case did not respond (not coded).
[b] 8 cases stated they wanted 3–4 children and these were coded as 3; 3 cases did not respond (not coded).

116

considerable education or women with secondary education. Age does not seem to be relevant. By creating the various categories shown and collapsing them to produce the appearance of convincing findings, we force conclusions because we have focused on the significance of the numbers in each cell rather than worrying about how the numbers were placed in the cells. If we claim that poorly educated women and men of all ages in one South American country express a desire for few children, we induce speculation on why this could occur, since the facts in other countries are the opposite.

The speculation about adults with little education leads to further examination of possible relevant variables in the case of Argentine fertility. Can significant correlations be found that would "lock in" a particular conclusion about the attitudes of Argentines with little educa-

TABLE 1A.   IDEAL FAMILY SIZE BY AGE AND EDUCATION

| | Number of Respondents in Each Age/Education Category | | | | | | |
| Ideal Family Size | Primary or Less | | Some Secondary or Completed | | Some University or Completed | | Totals |
	30 or Less	Over 30	30 or Less	Over 30	30 or Less	Over 30	
Men[a]							
3 children or fewer	6	40	2	11	—	10	69
4 or more children	1	19	1	2	—	7	30
							—
							99
Women[b]							
3 children or fewer	15	61	6	11	1	3	97
4 or more children	4	32	3	12	—	1	52
							—
							149

[a] 7 cases stated they wanted 3–4 children and these were coded as 3; 1 case did not respond.

[b] 8 cases stated they wanted 3–4 children and these were coded as 3; 3 cases did not respond.

tion? The gross demographic data on Argentina suggest that the present findings are not unusual because the country has had a low fertility rate for some time. We could reason that the country's high literacy rate, despite variations in formal education, may mean that more persons are exposed to attitudes favoring small families. (The birth rate for Argentina in 1960 was approximately 22 per 1000 of the total population—one of the lowest in Latin America.) The central issue is whether actual and desired family size should be related to education level, to the sex of the respondent, or to age. The finding of a correlation between education and family size, or church attendance and family size, or income and family size, does not prove that the researcher has examined the everyday conditions and experiences of family life, or that he has ascertained how decisions are made or avoided. Instead, all possible interpretations of the researcher's question–answer strategy are explored, to code materials that will yield the largest number of correlations. When a correlation that seems fairly high emerges, the researcher begins to advance ad hoc explanations of the phenomenon, concluding that differential fertility can be explained as evidenced by the correlation.

Presupposed in the researcher's designation of variables are some parallel ideas about what motivates people to engage in different types of action. In Latin America, low income, low education, frequent church attendance, and strong kinship ties are considered by the researcher to be conducive to high fertility. The reasons for claiming that correlations between actual family size and the foregoing "variables" imply a causal nexus must be checked in specific populations. An additional assumption might be that differential fertility can be attributed to organized belief systems. Thus a poorly educated man or woman with strong kinship ties, low income, and frequent church attendance would be expected to possess a belief system that emphasizes a large family size; but the same belief system would not link smaller families to individual comforts and greater national economic productivity, as suggested by studies cited in earlier chapters. With more education, higher income, and greater secularization of religious beliefs in a context of fewer kinship ties, the researcher's argument suggests, there emerges an instrumental belief system that is motivated to maximize individual comforts and opportunities for the parents and their offspring. But the study of everyday reasoning and belief systems, or how they change, is not viewed as basic to the traditional researcher's interpretation of tabulated "data" used for analysis.

The instrumental belief system or "modern man" notion I have barely outlined is linked to ideas about economic development, enlightened social values, democracy, equality, and the like. Many demographic studies employ such concepts in their survey studies of fertility, although they do not engage in independent studies of the same formulations in Western and non-Western belief systems. My interest is not in revealing how differential fertility is to be explained within a particular ideological framework; rather, I seek to learn how claims to knowledge formulated within all ideological perspectives or belief systems must satisfy normative accounts constructed from our situated experiences.

Additional tables are presented next to reveal further details relating to fertility and family planning. Table 2 gives the respective religions of the men and women in each respondent's family. Aside from noting the Catholic majority, there is little to add: Argentina is a Catholic country with a low birth rate. Table 2A offers something to talk about because the low rate of church attendance is ambiguous. The question asked was

TABLE 2.   RELIGION OF RESPONDENT'S FAMILY

Religion	Men	Women	Total
Catholic	78	124	202
Protestant	4	9	13
Other Christian religions	2	5	7
Jewish	6	8	14
Other	—	2	2
None	9	4	13
No information	1	—	1
Total	100	152	252

TABLE 2A.   CHURCH ATTENDANCE BY SEX OF RESPONDENT[a]

Attends Church	Men	Women	Total
Once a month or more	26	68	94
Irregularly or not at all	34	60	94
Never	28	19	47
Not religious	11	3	14
Total	99	150	249

[a] 3 cases (1 male and 2 women) were not coded because their responses were ambiguous.

"How often do you attend (go to) church during the month?" The responses varied considerably, making it difficult to create numerical differences. I preferred not to use a fixed-choice question, which would have forced respondents to resolve their doubts about attendance. The open-ended question selected permitted the interviewer to explore the possible ambiguities of the respondents' church attendance. Although Table 2A suggests that less than half the sample attend church regularly, the category we used—"goes once or more each month"—is not a strong indication of regularity. But the traditional survey research strategy is to build up a consistent argument, making it feasible to link church attendance figures to the desire for fewer children.

The distribution of desired family size (Table 3) suggests some of the difficulties of coding "data" on church attendance when the respondents have been limited to certain answers by the researcher's desire to obtain clear numerical differences. We observe that 78 respondents were ambivalent about how many children they desired. Table 3 is complicated to read, but it seems to indicate that often more children were desired than were actually borne. The respondents who claim to be more regular in their church attendance seem to have a slight tendency to want more children than they have. The tendency would probably be more noticeable if I had coded "up" instead of "down" when the number desired was expressed as 1–2 or 3–4. The reader might ask whether age were perhaps a factor here. If the sample were young, the possibility of more children would render Table 3 misleading. Before turning to this issue, let us consider Tables 3A, 3B, 3C, and 3D, which indicate that among the males church attendance has no clear relationship with a desire to have more children. The tendency to want more children is more closely associated with frequency of church attendance among women. The traditional assumption here is that church attendance signifies stronger religious commitments (Catholics), less likelihood of attitudes favoring the restriction of family size, and more likelihood of negative views about the use of contraceptives. But the family size desired is not particularly large, even among the women in the sample. If we were to combine the apparent desire among women for small families with the "collapsed" results in Table 3B and the actual family size of Tables 3C and 3D, we might conclude that our sample of Argentines is not very religious and that this has perhaps influenced their low fertility rate and their relatively low desire for large families. We could add additional "variables" such as rural–urban differences, noting that most of the people in the sample (Table 3, Chapter 4) were born in an urban area and that inasmuch as

TABLE 3. IDEAL FAMILY SIZE (NUMBER OF CHILDREN) BY CHURCH ATTENDANCE AND ACTUAL FAMILY SIZE

Ideal Family Size[a,b,c]	Attends Church Once a Month or More — Actual Family Size						Does Not Attend Church or Attends Irregularly — Actual Family Size						Never Attends Church — Actual Family Size						Not Religious — Actual Family Size						Totals
	0	1	2	3	4	5+	0	1	2	3	4	5+	0	1	2	3	4	5+	0	1	2	3	4	5+	
Males																									
0	—	—	—	—	—	—	—	—	—	—	—	—	—	—	1	—	—	—	—	1	1	—	—	—	1
1	—	1	—	—	—	—	—	1	1	—	—	—	—	1	1	—	—	—	—	1	1	2	—	—	7
2	—	—	2	2	—	—	2	6	6	2	—	1	4	3	5	1	—	—	—	1	2	2	—	—	39
3	1	2	4	1	3	1	—	5	1	1	—	1	—	3	3	1	—	—	—	—	—	—	—	—	24
4	—	—	1	1	—	2	2	1	3	2	1	—	1	—	2	1	1	—	—	—	—	1	—	—	16
5+	—	1	1	—	—	—	1	1	—	—	1	—	1	—	1	1	—	—	—	—	—	1	—	—	12
																									99
Females																									
0	—	—	—	—	—	—	—	—	—	—	—	—	—	—	—	—	—	—	—	—	—	—	—	—	—
1	—	2	—	—	—	1	—	1	—	—	—	—	—	1	—	—	—	—	—	—	—	—	—	—	3
2	3	4	5	1	—	1	2	14	3	2	—	1	4	2	2	—	—	—	—	1	—	—	—	—	48
3	—	5	7	7	1	5	3	6	3	1	—	2	1	1	4	—	1	—	—	—	—	—	—	—	44
4	3	3	8	1	1	4	2	1	3	1	2	1	—	2	3	1	1	—	—	1	—	—	—	—	37
5+	—	2	2	—	—	4	1	1	—	1	1	1	—	—	—	—	—	—	—	—	—	—	—	—	12
																									144

[a] Ideal family size not clear—6 female cases not coded.
[b] Unclear information on church attendance for: one male with ideal size and actual size as 2, one female with ideal size of 2 and actual size of 3, and one female with ideal size of 4 and actual size of 5.
[c] Brief tabulation of ideal family size (IFS) as coded for 78 cases.

IFS	Coded as	Males	Females
1-2	1	4	2
2-3	2	13	21
3-4	3	7	12
4-5	4	6	9
2-4	3	2	0
4-6	5	1	0
2-3 or 4-5	2	1	—

TABLE 3A.   IDEAL FAMILY SIZE (NUMBER OF CHILDREN) BY CHURCH ATTENDANCE
AND SEX OF RESPONDENT

Ideal Family Size	Attends Once a Month or More	Attends Irregularly or Does not Attend	Never Attends Church	Not Religious[b]	Totals
Males					
0	—	—	1	—	1
1	1	1	2	3	7
2	4	17	13	5	39
3	9	7	7	2	24
4	7	5	4	—	16
5+	2	6	3	1	12
					99
Females[a]					
0	—	—	—	—	—
1	2	1	—	—	3
2	14	27	6	1	48
3	19	18	6	1	44
4	21	9	7	—	37
5+	8	4	—	—	12
					144

[a] Ideal family size not clear—6 cases not coded.
[b] Unclear information on church attendance for one male (ideal = 2; actual = 2);
one female (ideal = 2; actual = 3); and one female (ideal = 4; actual 5+).

they all live in the highly urbanized area of Buenos Aires, lower fertility and a desire for smaller families should be expected. But "variables" like urbanization are too comprehensive and do not identify the characteristics of urban living that lead to small families or the desire for small families. We can refer to the crowded conditions of urban areas—and Buenos Aires certainly fits this image, for housing is hard to find and marriage is often delayed for years until a couple in the lower middle or middle class can find an apartment. But how these persons reason about such decisions is not clear, nor is it clear what logic working-class families use in considering their housing situations before deciding (by fiat?) on the number of children they will have.

If we wanted to be consistent with the survey research approach to

TABLE 3B.   IDEAL FAMILY SIZE[a] (NUMBER OF CHILDREN) BY CHURCH ATTENDANCE[b] (COLLAPSED VERSION)

Ideal Family Size	Attends Regularly Once or More Each Month	Attends Irregularly or Not at All	Not Religious	Totals
Males				
0	—	1	—	1
1	1	3	3	7
2	4	30	5	39
3	8	14	2	24
4	7	9	—	16
5+	2	9	1	12
				—
				99
Females				
0	—	—	—	1
1	2	1	—	3
2	14	33	1	48
3	19	24	1	44
4	21	16	—	37
5+	8	4	—	12
				—
				144

[a] Ideal family size not clear—6 female cases.
[b] Poor information on church attendance—3 cases (1 male and 2 females).

fertility, we would conclude that Buenos Aires seems to fit a broad structural pattern described by social scientists as peculiar to industrialized sectors of the western world: crowded urban conditions and secular attitudes, which result in an apparent "desire" for smaller families.

Within a traditional analysis, the age of the respondents cannot be ignored. Table 4 indicates that most of these queried who wanted larger families were 41 years of age or older, hence not likely to have more children. This observation is not too important, since most of our sample was in the 41 years and over age group. Additional information on desired family size by age of respondent at the time of the interview suggests that those who were ambivalent about the number of children desired (for which I coded down) were not the younger members of the sample but were primarily respondents who were not likely to have more

TABLE 3C.   ACTUAL FAMILY SIZE BY CHURCH ATTENDANCE[a]

Actual Family Size	Attends Once a Month or More	Attends Irregularly or Not at All	Never Attends Church	Not Religious	Totals
Males					
0	1	5	6	1	
1	4	13	7	2	
2	8	10	13	3	
3	3	5	3	5	
4	3	2	1	—	
5+	3	1	—	—	
	22	36	30	11	99
Females					
0	6	8	1	1	
1	17	24	7	1	
2	23	17	10	—	
3	10	4	1	—	
4	1	3	1	—	
5+	11	4	—	—	
	68	60	20	2	150

[a] No information on church attendance—3 cases (1 male and 2 female).

children. In some of the younger couples, conflict between husband and wife is suggested. It is possible to argue that the women in the sample wanted more children (although Argentine fertility would not be very high even if these desires were realized). But the condensed information on ideal family size by age at interview and actual family size, provided by Table 4A suggests how difficult it is to pinpoint crude yet recordable discrepancies between the preferences of husband and wife. Many families do not agree about how many children they want, and these differences are hard to specify in tables.

Tables 4B and 4C provide additional bases for speculation. For the older respondents, the discrepancy between desired family size and actual family size can be accounted for as a nostalgic, retrospective rereading of each respondent's married life. The interview setting gave the older respondents an occasion for reviewing the past and making abstract replies that conveniently did away with the possibility of recovering

TABLE 3D.   ACTUAL FAMILY SIZE BY CHURCH ATTENDANCE[a] (COLLAPSED VERSION)

Actual Family Size	Attends Regularly Once or More Each Month	Attends Irregularly or Not at All	Not Religious	Totals
Males				
0	1	11	1	
1	4	20	2	
2	8	23	3	
3	3	8	5	
4	3	3	—	
5+	3	1	—	
	22	66	11	99
Females				
0	6	9	1	
1	17	31	1	
2	23	27	1	
3	10	5	—	
4	1	4	—	
5+	11	4	—	
	68	80	2	150

[a] No information on church attendance—3 cases (1 male and 2 female).

day-to-day details. These expressed desires tell us nothing about the lived experiences of the earlier years, and we probably would not be justified in maintaining that the desires expressed at the time of the interviews represent "real" events. There is a lack of articulation between the desires expressed during the interview and the experiences that may have been connected to the actual family situations throughout the marriage. Whatever is "actual" about the present level of fertility in a family has its own unexplicated history.

To view "actual" fertility, recorded at different points in real time, as a series of localized decisions or fortuitous arrangements may appear to be unreasonable to the traditional sociological researcher or population expert. After all, the researcher presumes that contrasting distributions within regions of a country or between different countries (with controls for urbanization, religion, chuch attendance, income, education, industrialization, attitudes toward desired family size, use of contraceptives, etc.) serve to indicate such "real" causal forces as an instrumental belief

TABLE 4. IDEAL FAMILY SIZE (NUMBER OF CHILDREN) BY AGE AT INTERVIEW AND ACTUAL FAMILY SIZE

	Age at Interview																														Totals
	21–25						26–30						31–35						36–40						41+						
Ideal Family Size[a]	0	1	2	3	4	5+	0	1	2	3	4	5+	0	1	2	3	4	5+	0	1	2	3	4	5+	0	1	2	3	4	5+	
Males																															
0	—	—	—	—	—	—	—	—	—	—	—	—	—	—	—	—	—	—	—	—	—	—	—	—	—	1	—	—	—	—	
1	—	1	1	—	—	—	—	1	1	—	—	—	—	2	2	—	—	—	1	1	2	—	—	—	3	5	9	3	—	1	
2	—	1	1	—	—	—	—	1	1	—	—	—	—	2	2	—	—	—	—	2	2	—	—	—	1	7	6	4	—	1	
3	—	—	1	—	—	—	—	1	1	—	—	—	—	—	—	—	—	—	—	1	1	1	—	—	2	—	2	2	5	1	
4	1	—	—	—	—	—	—	1	1	—	—	—	—	1	—	—	—	—	—	1	1	—	—	—	2	2	3	2	1	—	
5+	—	1	—	—	—	—	1	—	—	—	—	—	—	1	—	—	—	—	—	1	—	—	—	1	2	3	—	—	—	—	100
Females																															
0	—	—	—	—	—	—	—	—	—	—	—	—	—	—	—	—	—	—	—	—	—	—	—	—	—	1	—	—	—	—	
1	2	3	—	—	—	—	—	2	—	—	—	—	—	1	4	—	—	—	—	3	3	2	—	—	2	11	8	2	—	2	
2	—	1	1	—	—	—	—	3	2	—	—	—	1	3	3	3	—	—	1	1	2	—	—	—	3	3	10	2	1	1	
3	—	1	1	—	—	—	—	2	4	1	—	—	1	3	1	—	—	1	1	5	2	1	1	1	3	3	4	1	3	5	
4	—	1	3	—	—	—	—	2	1	—	—	—	2	1	—	—	—	—	—	—	—	1	—	1	—	2	2	—	1	3	
5+	—	—	—	—	—	—	1	—	—	—	—	—	—	1	—	—	—	—	—	—	—	—	—	2	—	2	2	1	—	3	145

a Seven cases not recorded: no information on ideal family size—6 female cases; one woman, age 18, ideal 2 children, has 1. One male, age 57, ideal 2–3 or 4–5 children, has 7, coded as ideal = 2.

TABLE 4A.   ADDITIONAL INFORMATION ON TABLE 4

Ideal Family Size	Age[a]	
	Males	Females
1–2 (coded as 1)	28, 40, 54, 66	29, 47
2–3 (coded as 2)	23 (wife wants 4), 29, 34, 38, 38 (wife wants 4, have 2), 39, 40, 44, 49, 56, 58, 58, 65 (wife is 61, wanted 5, have 1)	21, 21, 28, 32, 33, 36, 36, 38, 39, 39, 43 (husband wanted 1), 45, 46, 48, 51, 52, 52 (husband wanted 4–5, have 3), 54, 56, 57, 59
3–4 (coded as 3)	38, 44, 47, 65, 66, 66, 72	28, 30 (husband is 31, wants 2, have 1), 30, 33, 34, 35, 42, 44 (husband wanted 2, have 2), 48 (husband wanted 8), 49, 56 (husband wanted 2, have 2)
4–5 (coded as 4)	22, 36, 43, 51, 63, 68	23 (husband wants 3, have 2), 28, 30, 36, 42, 42, 55 (husband desired 2–3), 56, 68
5–6 (coded as 5)	42, 51 (wife wanted 2, have 2)	28 (married at 25, husband wants 2, have 0), 48, 58 (husband wanted 3, have 1)
6–7 (coded as 6)	—	47 (husband wanted 3, have 5)
7–8 (coded as 7)	—	76 (has 5)
2–4 (coded as 3)	45, 55 (wife is 59, wanted 2–3, have 2)	—
4–6 (coded as 5)	43 (wife is 39, wanted 6, have 5)	—

[a] Age differences between husband and wife in four families:
   wife age 26 wants 1, has 1; husband is 30, wants 3
   wife age 22 wants 4, has 1; husband is 21, wants 2
   wife age 42 wants 4–5, has 2; husband is 37, wants 5
   wife age 38 wants 2, has 2; husband is 40, wants 0

TABLE 4B   IDEAL FAMILY SIZE (NUMBER OF CHILDREN) BY AGE AT INTERVIEW

Ideal Family Size[a]	Age at Interview					Totals
	21–25	26–30	31–35	36–40	41+	
Males[b, c]						
0	—	—	—	—	1	1
1	—	2	—	1	4	7
2	2	3	7	7	21	40
3	—	2	1	2	19	24
4	1	—	—	3	12	16
5+	—	—	1	1	10	12
						100
Females[d, e]						
0	—	—	—	—	—	—
1	—	2	—	—	1	3
2	6	3	5	9	25	48
3	3	7	11	4	19	44
4	4	3	3	9	19	37
5+	—	1	1	2	8	12
						145

[a] No information on ideal family size—6 cases not coded.
[b] Total males; ages 21–40: 33; total age 41+: 67.
[c] One male, age 57, ideal 2–3 or 4–5 children, has 7, recorded as 2.
[d] Total females, ages 21–40; 73; total age 41+: 72.
[e] One woman, age 18, ideal 2 children, has 1, not recorded.

system at work, producing the distributional differences. I have stressed that the conditions for obtaining information influence directly what we will call "data" and that when these conditions remain unexamined and daily family living is ignored, explanations of the causes of fertility are difficult to accept. The "clarity" of the tables is only apparent when the reader is not encumbered with basic "data" giving the complicated details of how the interview was accomplished and how the answers were coded.

But the population expert needs to know whether age at interview is producing an effect on church attendance. If the sample is top-heavy with older respondents, cross-tabulating desired family size with church attendance would not reveal the influence of age on church attendance. The

TABLE 4C. ACTUAL FAMILY SIZE (NUMBER OF CHILDREN) BY AGE AT INTERVIEW[a]

	Age at Interview					
Actual Family Size	21–25	26–30	31–35	36–40	41+	Totals
Males						
0	1	2	1	1	8	13
1	1	3	3	3	17	27
2	1	2	3	6	22	34
3	—	—	2	3	11	16
4	—	—	—	—	6	6
5+	—	—	—	1	3	4
						100
Females						
0	2	1	3	2	8	16
1	5	9	5	6	24	49
2	3	5	8	10	24	50
3	1	1	4	4	5	15
4	—	—	—	1	4	5
5+	—	—	1	4	11	16
						151

[a] One woman, age 18, has 1 child, not recorded.

population expert must determine whether the younger respondents are attending church as often as or less often than older respondents. Any number of arguments could then be advanced about the implications of more or less attendance for forecasting fertility trends. Table 5 suggests that church attendance remains higher for older respondents, but primarily for the women in the sample. Thus we could argue that our small sample of urban Argentines is not very religious and that even those who are religious seem to be restricting their fertility behavior to an extent that contrasts sharply with the rest of Latin America. We could conclude that our small sample from Buenos Aires reflects the national picture of small family size and that even if desired family sizes were reached, the fertility rate would not be increased appreciably.

One's interpretation of survey results depends on the researcher's strategy for convincing the reader: does he seek a detailed cross-tabulation of results, or does he allow the reader to make inferences from the raw

TABLE 5.   CHURCH ATTENDANCE BY AGE AT INTERVIEW

Church Attendance	Age at Interview					Totals
	21–25	26–30	31–35	36–40	41+	
Males[a]						
Attends regularly once or more each month	—	—	1	1	20	22
Attends irregularly or not at all	3	5	6	12	40	66
Not religious	—	2	2	1	6	11
						99
Females[b,c]						
Attends regularly once or more each month	5	6	9	8	40	68
Attends irregularly or not at all	8	10	10	15	36	79
Not religious	—	1	—	—	1	2
						149

[a] One male, age 63, no information on church attendance.
[b] One female, age 18, does not attend church—not recorded.
[c] One female, age 52, no information on church attendance; one female, age 74, no information on church attendance.

materials. A few studies (Stycos 1955; Blake 1961) have used tables as a point of departure for revealing elements of contextual responses by the use of direct quotations from the subjects. The details provided by the quotations give the reader a sense of depth not captured by demographic tables; but these quoted fragments can also be misleading because the reader is not exposed to the interactional context within which the interview was negotiated. The direct quotations do not examine the language used by interviewer and respondent; moreover, they are presumed to be obvious, direct lines of communication to feelings or attitudes, which the researcher treats as context-free conditions for describing differential fertility.

Tables on Family Size and the Use of Contraceptives. If the sample tabulation indicates a desire for relatively small families and respondents report they have small families, it is traditionally appropriate to ask whether our respondents achieved small families because of a familiarity with contraceptives. Table 6 suggests that the members of the sample were familiar with contraceptives. During our interviews in Buenos Aires, posing questions about contraceptives created difficulties. Respondents seemed to want to answer our questions quickly and to move on to a presumably less bothersome subject. In Table 7 only a few of the cases are listed as having reported vague answers. One problem was that if we asked people to name all known methods of contraception, many subjects (often the less educated) seemed to be embarrassed, and they began to hesitate or stammer. This evident discomfort might have been

TABLE 6.   KNOWLEDGE OF CONTRACEPTIVES BY SEX OF RESPONDENT

Knowledge of Contraceptives	Men[a]	Women
Has heard of one or more methods	95	148
Has not heard of modern methods	2	4
Total	97	152

[a] No information on two men. One male respondent could not be asked about contraceptives because of interference by the wife.

TABLE 7.   KNOWLEDGE OF EACH CONTRACEPTIVE METHOD BY SEX OF RESPONDENT

Method	Men[a]	Women[b]
Condom	95	140
Douche	26	38
Foam tablets	7	6
Diaphragm	14	20
Withdrawal	42	65
Pill	11	11
Intrauterine device	16	26
Button	19	25
Jelly	27	32
Rhythm	12	33

[a] No information on 3 men. One response is vague; another, according to the coder, did not respond because of the wife's interference.
[b] No information on 4 women; 5 women with vague or ambiguous responses.

due to unfamiliarity with the nomenclature the respondent thought was used normally by others, or to ignorance of methods in general. The respondent might have felt he or she was being tested about his education or intelligence. If the interviewer showed a card listing various methods or named each method, asking the respondent to indicate those he "knew," we would still have trouble validating the answers because we could never determine what the respondent knew before we furnished a set of possible answers to our question. To ask how each method works raises the issue of his education or intelligence again. The materials in Table 7 appear more impressive than we have a right to expect, although perhaps a sample or population that has maintained such low fertility rates for as long as the Argentine sample, might be expected to have considerable knowledge about methods of contraception.

Consider the complications encountered in discussing the details of knowledge and use of contraceptives. Attempts to ascertain which member of a couple used contraceptives and with what frequency proved difficult, as did attempts to learn how subjects initially heard about contraceptives. Details of their experiments with different methods were very hard to secure, as were estimates of the influence (or lack of it) of such experiences on family planning. Our approach was to avoid mentioning specific methods until we were satisfied that the subject could not tell us anything of value in response to the questions we asked. In some cases the interviewers were instructed to mention one or two methods "in vague terms." A serious problem was encountered when we tried to link the acquisition of information about the use of contraceptives with occasions of pregnancy. Our interview procedures were designed to trace the history of the acquisition of information on contraceptives, but the respondents did not cooperate readily. Except for a few cases in which the interviewers seemed to establish a relationship that permitted more extensive probes, the respondents only gave brief answers.

Continuing our traditional analysis, we can use Table 8 to indicate that most of the sample seems to approve of the use of contraceptives, regardless of desired family size or sex of the respondent. Table 9 merely reinforces this view. The respondents were asked whether they approved of others using contraceptives, and most of those who were ambivalent or disapproved for themselves did not seem to object to others using contraceptive methods.

When a "positive attitude" toward limiting family size was contrasted with social class, it appeared that the number of women approving

TABLE 8. ATTITUDES TOWARD THE LIMITATION OF FAMILY SIZE BY SEX OF RESPONDENT

Attitude Toward Limiting Family Size	Total Sample		Cases Expressing an Ideal Family Size of 3 or Fewer Children		Cases Expressing an Ideal Family Size of 4 or More Children	
	Men[a]	Women[b]	Men	Women	Men	Women
Approve	69	108	57	86	12	22
Ambivalent	21	28	16	17	5	11
Object	9	12	6	4	3	8
Total	99	148	79	107	20	41

[a] No information for one male respondent.

[b] Four women were listed as ambiguous ("it depends," "I'm not sure") in their responses, according to the coder.

TABLE 9. ATTITUDES TOWARD THE USE OF CONTRACEPTIVES BY OTHERS

Attitude	Men[a]	Women[b]
Yes, in general, and for economic reasons	89	136
Yes, but only for health reasons	5	10
No, despite endangering the mother's health	—	—
No, in general	3	2
Don't know	1	3
Total	98	151

[a] No information on one male case; another answered "it depends on one's conscience"; according to coder.

[b] No information on one female case; another allowed for both economic and health reasons in limiting family size and was scored as "economic."

limitation was distributed fairly uniformly over the different socioeconomic levels. Table 10 appears to show that women approve of limiting family size, regardless of social class and the number of children they desire. From Table 11, which supplies additional details about the women of our sample, it appears that most of the women, regardless of age, are in favor of limiting family size. Nor does the number of children in the family

TABLE 10.   ATTITUDES TOWARD LIMITING FAMILY SIZE BY FEMALE RESPONDENTS AND SOCIOECONOMIC STATUS

Socioeconomic Status[a]	Approve Limitation[b]	Approve Limitation and Consider Ideal Family Size to be 3 or Fewer Children
Low		
1–2	36	26
3	38	27
4–5	34	25
High		
6–7	10	6
Total	118	84

[a] As grouped in Germani's sample (Table 2, Chapter 4).
[b] No information on Socioeconomic status for two women approving limitation.

or the number of years since the last pregnancy seem to make much difference with respect to attitudes toward limiting family size. In Table 12 most members of the sample are coded as expressing a favorable attitude toward limiting family size, despite having fewer children than they consider ideal.

The tables presented thus far would allow us to assemble evidence in support of the traditional arguments that small families are desired in Argentina and that practical adherence to such attitudes is evidenced by the small size of actual families. Additional speculative arguments can be made by noting that the families interviewed are underproducing with respect to desired family size, regardless of sex, age, social class, or number of years since a woman's last pregnancy. We could add that "other factors" associated with urban living are probably influencing the underproduction (e.g., the lack of housing in Buenos Aires, the desire on the part of many women to pursue occupational careers, and the desire for material objects and leisure activities). We could add other abstract arguments that would link low fertility to a widespread cynicism about the economic instability in Argentina and a general malaise associated with political instability and corruption.

To pursue the traditional argument further, the reader could ask how Argentines implement their desires for smaller families. Tables 13 through 17 suggest that most of the sample members have discussed the use of contraceptives (but this assumption is compromised by the vague-

TABLE 11. WOMEN'S ATTITUDES TOWARD THE LIMITATION OF FAMILY SIZE BY AGE, NUMBER OF LIVING CHILDREN, AND NUMBER OF YEARS SINCE LAST PREGNANCY

Characteristics	Approve of Limitation	Object or Are Ambivalent About Limitation	Totals
Age			
30 or less	26	4	30
Over 30	92	30	122
			152
Total living children			
None	16	4	20
1–2	82	13	95
3	12	3	15
4 or more	11	10	21
			151[a]
Years since last pregnancy			
Pregnant	8	3	11
0–1	19	6	25
2–3	11	3	14
4–5	8	1	9
6 or more	65	20	85
Does not apply	6	2	8
			152

[a] No information for one case.

ness of the questions) and that most responses seem to be consistent within each couple with respect to claims to having discussed the issue together. The practice of limiting family size seems clear in Table 15— most respondents reported having used one or more methods for limiting family size, particularly those persons desiring three or fewer children. Table 15 poses a problem, since not all the women indicating a preference for three or fewer children could be coded because of the interviewer's lack of information about actual use of contraceptive methods. The women desiring smaller families seemed to be actively using some form of contraception (Table 16), but so were women who desired larger families. Most of the women claimed to use some form of contraceptive.

TABLE 12.   ATTITUDE TOWARD LIMITING FAMILY SIZE BY FEMALE RESPONDENTS BY IDEAL VERSUS ACTUAL FAMILY SIZE

Family Size	Approve of Limitation	Ambivalent About or Object to Limitation
Respondent has fewer children than ideal		
2 less	46	15
1 less	43	7
Actual children equals ideal	26	5
More children than ideal		
1 more	1	—
2 more	1	—
3–4 more	1	2
5–8 more	1	1
Total	117	31

[a] 3 cases not recorded; no information on 2 females.

TABLE 13.   COMMUNICATION BETWEEN SPOUSES ABOUT THE USE OF CONTRACEPTIVES

Discussion with Spouse[a]	Men	Women
Yes	64	106
No	28	39
Total	92	145

[a] 8 men and 7 women were not coded for lack of information.

Table 17 reports on attitudes toward contraceptive use among those who know the methods and who approve of limiting a family to three children or fewer. This table is not conclusive, however, because in a great many cases the interviewer indicated "no information"—a rather unfortunate "response," particularly since it was so difficult to induce respondents to talk about their experiences or knowledge.

Concluding Remarks.   In using a questionnaire with traditional fixed-choice questions, the interviewer might simply repeat a question three times and go on to the next, without knowing whether the respondent had understood the syntax of the question, much less the terms employed. Questionnaires are designed for "educated" respondents; but what "edu-

TABLE 14. COMPARISON OF COUPLES WHO DISCUSSED THE USE OF CONTRACEPTIVES WITH THEIR SPOUSES

Type of Response	Frequency
Both said yes	49
Both said no	14
Wife said yes, husband no	7
Husband said yes, wife no	7
No information for both	2
No information for one spouse	3
	—
Total couples	82

TABLE 15. RESPONDENTS REPORTING THE USE OR NONUSE OF CONTRACEPTIVES BY SEX AND THOSE APPROVING OF A SMALL FAMILY (3 CHILDREN OR FEWER) (EXCLUDING ABSTINENCE AND ABORTIONS AS CONCTRACEPTIVE METHODS)

	Those Approving of Small Family (3 Children or Fewer)		Remainder of Sample	
Reported Practice	Men	Women	Men	Women
Has used one or more methods	54	64	25	48
Has never used any method	1	2	15	30
Total[a]	55	66	40	78

[a] Poor information for 5 men and 8 women.

cation" entails is never clear, and the same questionnaire will also be used for "uneducated" respondents, with the possible modification of allowing interviewers to take unspecified liberties in explaining the questions. A central issue in the study of family planning and the use of contraceptives is deciding how to obtain and interpret information. The interviewer's written materials assume that each set of answers incorporates the respondent's understanding of the researcher's intentions. The standard questionnaire study does not address the issues of the interviewer's interpretation of the respondent's answer and the respondent's understanding of the researcher's intentions. The researcher must communicate with a respondent whose interest in and knowledge of the

TABLE 16.   TYPE OF CONTRACEPTION USED BY WOMEN APPROVING FAMILY
LIMITATION AND WANTING A SMALL FAMILY (3 CHILDREN OR FEWER)

Type of Method Used	Women Who Approve of Limiting Family Size (Ideal of 3 Children or Fewer)	Rest of Sample
Chemical–mechanical	36	18
Withdrawal	25	18
Abstinence	11	8
Total[a]	72	44

[a] Unclear information on 4 women.

TABLE 17.   ATTITUDES TOWARD PARTICULAR CONTRACEPTIVE METHODS BY MEN
AND WOMEN CLAIMING KNOWLEDGE OF THE METHODS AND APPROVING
OF CONTRACEPTIVES AND SMALL FAMILIES (3 CHILDREN OR FEWER)

Indicated Attitude by Method	Men	Women
Douche		
Approve	11	11
Ambivalent	—	2
Object	3	4
No information	46	60
Condom		
Approve	46	53
Ambivalent	—	4
Object	13	14
No information	1	6
Withdrawal		
Approve	27	40
Ambivalent	1	1
Object	8	2
No information	23	35

study may be minimal—a respondent whose awareness of issues and ability to receive questions and formulate answers may be quite limited.

"Interpretation" of Tables 1 and 1A (ideal family size by age and education) may appear to be self-evident, but determining the level of education is ambiguous because of the questions used, despite the attempt to obtain additional information. We began by asking if the

respondent had been able to attend school (*¿Pudo Ud. ir a la escuela?*)
and what type of school he had attended—state, private, or religious
(*¿A qué tipo de escuela fue? ¿Del estado, privada, religioso, o no?*) . We
asked where the schools were located (*¿Dónde estaba ubicada la escuela?*) ,
the level of schooling achieved (*¿Hasta qué nivel escolar llegó?*), and
whether the respondent had been exposed to such non-academic subjects
as dressmaking or typing (*¿Estudió alguna otra cosa? ¿Como corte y
confección, dactilografía?*). We wanted to gain a general idea of the kind
of education achieved and of its quality in terms of whether the
school was in a rural area, whether it was state supported, private,
and so forth. Answers were frequently vague or very brief. The
questions often seemed to be a source of embarrassment to the respondents. It is very difficult to allege that the categories in Tables 1 and 1A
present degrees of sophistication or indicate how respondents managed
their everyday lives. We must resign ourselves to the realization that
establishing cutoff points (e.g., "no education," "primary education," or
"secondary education") means that we have only a vague sense of the
respondent's degree of "civilization" or knowledge; thus we cannot
accurately evaluate his ability to answer questions pertaining to the kind
of family desired or to ways of limiting family size. When we use such
categories as "primary incomplete" or "secondary incomplete," we can
never decide whether a particular respondent did poorly in school and
finally dropped out to work, whether he or she was forced to drop out
for economic reasons, or whether going through school meant very little
to the respondent. Thus when we cross-tabulate this "variable" of educational achievement with desired family size by age and sex, we are somehow presupposing that any correlation found will imply (*a*) that levels
of education orient a person's thinking toward family size in particular
ways and (*b*) that this orientation is affected by age and sex. The researcher merely asks that differences appear between cells in the tables.
With an "adequate" sample size and "appropriate" splits in the data, the
researcher can easily create an acceptable explanation for each table.

If we want to believe the tables we must ignore countless contingencies
requiring tacit decisions made by the interviewer and by the respondent
for the purpose of completing the interviewing and the coding of responses. We could conclude that the sample survey results just reported
suggest that Argentines approve of family planning and the practice of
limiting births. We could substantiate the appearance of Argentina's low
fertility by adding any number of related ethnographic details about the
scarcity of housing, the delays in marriage that are based on difficulties

in finding jobs and scarcity in housing, the relatively low cost of abortions, and a high level of urbanization and literacy. I reported only some of the tables that could have been assembled from the survey questionnaire to illustrate the brief description of fertility behavior in Argentina. Rather than present more tables, I have elected to reveal how a textual analysis of the interview materials contrasts with the tables.

In the study of human social behavior we depend on verbal question and answer exchanges for generating convincing accounts of our ideas and experiences and for making claims to knowledge. Hence we find it difficult (and risky, if we are tied to traditional surveys and census materials) to describe other verbal and nonverbal ways of communicating intentions, desires, and uncertainties. We are forced to imagine, and we must persuade the reader to imagine or to invent possible social settings; and we tacitly elaborate ethnographic settings to animate the tables we employ for claims to knowledge. The day-to-day settings we live in, and the simple or elaborate social routines that adults construct to avoid or encourage sexual activities are not studied as integral parts of human fertility behavior and family planning.

In the next chapter I examine interviews that are a mixture of verbatim notes and paraphrased reconstructions by the interviewers and consider how such materials can alter the textual analysis of questions and responses. An additional chapter focuses on changes in interpretation introduced by a tape-recorded interview. The next two chapters clarify the nature of fertility activities as situated events.

CHAPTER 8

TEXTUAL ANALYSIS OF INTERVIEW MATERIALS

Sexual Unions

ONE WIFE'S PERSPECTIVE. The interviews utilized many questions as probes, to aid in determining conditions of sexual relations between the spouses to find out whether sexual relations influenced the number of children desired and the number actually borne. The questions met with mixed success—occasional interviews produced interesting details, whereas in other cases the respondents seemed to attempt to satisfy the interviewer with a minimal "answer" in the hope that the topic would be dropped. In the tables presented, the coded cross-tabulations do not reveal these nuances in sexual relations between the spouses. The following case, taken at random from a table entry already discussed, represents the part of the sample indicating that more children were desired than had been borne. The wife had expressed a desire for three children, and the couple actually had one. The woman was 31 years old, she had had a primary education, and her life style could be described loosely as lower middle income. The language employed by the respondent seemed rather sophisticated to me, so I began examining the interviewer's remarks. I found that it had been difficult to obtain the interview because the respondent created many delays and excuses, although she had agreed to various appointments. The interviewer noted, however, that the woman was apologetic about the delays and remarked that her husband had been interviewed the night before by a male interviewer and that "he was made to (they made him) talk as never before in his life" ("*le hicieron hablar como nunca en su vida lo había hecho*"). The interview with the woman was described as intense, and the respondent was said to be attentive at all times, as well as "intelligent," "always alert," "quick to respond," and able "to get out of a tight spot gracefully" ("*salir airosa de un aprieto*"). The interviewer stated that the woman had acquired some refined mannerisms that would not ordinarily be associated with a person of her social standing. In accounting for this sophistication, the interviewer noted that the respondent had worked for many years in fashionable beauty salons in the center of Buenos Aires, where she had been able to pick up subtle interactional nuances. The woman's use of gestures was described as being natural and unaffected, and she used a broad vocabulary that seemed strange coming from her lips, because of her rather plain home and surroundings. The reader will notice that I have used a few ethnographic details to provide a "convincing" context for presenting a specific interpretation of the interview materials. My choice of particulars structures the interpretation I regard as plausible.

The questions began with the issue of discussions between the husband and wife about sexual relations. (The Spanish version is in the Appendix at the close of the chapter.)

1. INTERVIEWER. On some occasions do you talk with your husband about sexual relations? (FA 76 MU 163-31)
   RESPONDENT. Yes.
   INTERVIEWER. What types of things do you talk about? (163-31a)
   RESPONDENT. Within sensual matters, we say that for my husband, the bed represents 95% of the marriage, while for me only 5% ["many smiles" by respondent is reported by interviewer]. For me it is a complementary activity; I can't imagine (understand) how for some women everything gets resolved in bed. For my part, if everything else goes poorly, if I argue with my husband if there are fights, it can't be that everything is forgotten when one goes to bed with him. Don't you think so?

The respondent's remarks about the importance of "the bed" in her husband's idea of marriage (as opposed to her own) can offer a brief glimpse into some of the woman's thoughts about her marriage. These thoughts may reflect many encounters when routine or unusual arguments, disagreements, or discussions have made the prospect of going to bed rather dismal. The woman's remarks seem plausible, and the researcher may conclude that such comments have not been volunteered merely to cut off the interviewer. Although the interviewer did not press for more details, we can suggest in retrospect that the interviewer had missed an opportunity to obtain details on how everyday living affects sexual intercourse and perhaps indirectly a group's fertility rate. We can say that the woman's response is plausible or reasonable if we assume that her description of her attitudes about sex between her and her husband is "natural" in certain kinds of marriages (i.e., marriages in which the woman must wait for the husband to take the initiative, or in which the husband has been given or has insisted on making decisions about how sexual activities are to be managed).

If we had been asking fixed-choice questions, the issue of how language is used by the respondent would never be raised. Hence the issue of the language used would not provide additional information to assess our questions as relevant or superficial. But by looking at the woman's sophisticated language usage, we are able to return to her answer about sexual relations, adding that perhaps she is considerably more sophisticated than her husband and that her remarks about the unlikelihood of resolving everyday problems in bed point to a constant source of irritation that leads to strategies designed to thwart her husband's sexual desires. We could also argue that many of the woman's apparently "rich" remarks were nevertheless condensed responses designed to obscure certain issues. Or we could argue that the interview setting was not easy for the interviewer to manage because of the woman's sophistication at parrying questions, thus precluding additional probes by the interviewer. Perhaps the interviewer could not probe because she noticed particulars of intonation and facial glances or other warning gestures that could not be recorded.

The interviewer continued to question the respondent about the views of family size held by other couples and by the respondent. These questions were used because they were expected to produce details about how sexual relations between the spouses influenced family size.

2. INTERVIEWER. Do you know any married couples who do not have children? How many? (FA 76 MU 163-33)
   RESPONDENT. One.
   INTERVIEWER. Why don't they have children, what do you make of this? (163-33a)
   RESPONDENT. Because he didn't want to have any.
   INTERVIEWER. Let's take each family without children that you know: How did you find out? (163-33b)
   RESPONDENT. [No response. Interviewer indicates that the last answer was viewed as satisfying this question.]
   INTERVIEWER. Do you know a married couple that has one or two children? How many? (163-34)
   RESPONDENT. One, a sister.
   INTERVIEWER. Let's take married couples that you know with only one child,

what happened in the case of the first couple that you know of this type? (163-34a)

RESPONDENT. She wanted one, then she watched herself (looked after herself) and now she wants one but can't have one.

INTERVIEWER. (For each family with one or two children, ask:) "How did you come to know about the case of family X?" (163-34b)

RESPONDENT. [No response. Interviewer indicates that the last answer was viewed as satisfying this question.]

INTERVIEWER. In general, who do you think likes a large family, men or women? (163-35)

RESPONDENT. They both like them, the one and the other. [Two probes were to be used here, but the interviewer does not indicate what happened.]

INTERVIEWER. What do you think is the best (ideal) size for a family? (163-36)

RESPONDENT. Three children.

INTERVIEWER. (If the number given as the "best [ideal] size" is different from the actual number of children in the family of the respondent, ask:) "Why didn't you have three children?" (163-36a)

RESPONDENT. Because I have to wait a year and a half after (having) the daughter. The doctor recommended that I do this. I was left rather fragile (delicate).

INTERVIEWER. What is the ideal family (size) your husband prefers? (163-37)

RESPONDENT. Eleven children.

INTERVIEWER. How do you know that your husband feels (thinks) this way about this matter? (163-37a)

RESPONDENT. He adores kids; ever since he was a bachelor he said this.

There are several apparently unsatisfactory answers concerning couples known to have few children and the respondent's explanation of why these couples did not want more. The responses "because he didn't want to have any" and "she wanted one, then she watched herself (looked after herself), and now she wants one but can't have one" suggest either possible ignorance about details of the couples' use of contraceptives or a deliberate attempt to cut off further discussion.

The woman's reason for not having the three children she had indicated as ideal seemed to be plausible because it referred to a medical situation ("the doctor recommended . . ."), regarding which the interviewer asked no further questions. But note that the husband was said to want eleven children. It was also learned that he was four years younger than his wife and that (based on a later question not quoted here) the wife reported sexual intercourse with the husband as "very relative . . . once or twice a week." The wife, asked what kinds of things or activities the couple engaged in jointly, stated that they did virtually nothing together, that her husband was no help around the house, and that they were seldom together. These additional particulars can serve as a basis for considerable speculation about the discrepancy between the number of actual children and the number considered ideal. But what do we conclude if we look only at the "objective facts"? Do we conclude that some kind of planning is involved? Or do we suggest that the woman has been instrumental in reducing fertility because of apparent differences in her sexual appetite and that of her husband?

Other information from the interview can be linked to the tables in the preceding chapter. For example, the husband desired a large family while professing to have no religion, and the woman indicated that she went to church once in awhile. Do we conclude that professing no religion and wanting a large family is of significance? At the time of the interview, the couple had one daughter, age 8 months, and the woman had lost a newborn baby the year they were married. The woman did not sound eager to have more children, although this would have been possible. We might wonder whether her "delicate" condition and minimal ("5%") sexual appetite will influence her not to have additional children. How would these "factors" emerge in day-to-day family interaction?

In another part of the interview the respondent stated that she did not use contraceptives but did give herself a douche after intercourse. Yet she seemed to be familiar with a variety of contraceptives, including the diaphragm and the condom. She expressed her own dislike for using a contraceptive but stated that her sister and brother-in-law do use them. When she was asked if she would use contraceptives now, she responded affirmatively, but this marked the first time in the interview that she had said anything about their use. Her husband, she said, had not used contraceptives, and when asked whether she had discussed the use of contraceptives with her husband, she answered "no," adding that he knew he should be careful. When asked to summarize her husband's views on this issue, she stated "That he would like to be careful (use some kind of contraceptive [?] as protection), that he has the desire (to control himself) but cannot do it" (*Que a él le gustaría cuidarse, que tiene voluntad pero no puede hacerlo*"). Regarding the use of contraceptives, she also said "*no me lo tomé a pecho*"—she "didn't take it to heart." The implications of the remark that her husband wanted to use contraceptives but "cannot do it" are not clear. The woman noted that she, however, recognized the importance of contraceptives and learned more about them from her brother-in-law and sister. At one point the respondent used the expression that her husband "can't (stand) tolerate" (*"no lo puede tolerar"*) the use of contraceptives. Finally, she revealed that because of her delicate condition she could not become pregnant again for a time specified by her doctor, and that she sought to prevent pregnancy by the use of a douche.

There are several uses of language in the previous paragraphs that should be elaborated. For example, when the woman stated that her husband had the desire to use contraceptives but could not (somehow make himself) use them, she made an additional statement: asked her reaction to her husband's attitude on the use of contraceptives, she responded "I come out running; I do not make any problems for him, for whether my husband uses them or not, I understand that he has the desire to use it but cannot." (*"Salgo corriendo. No le hago problema, mi marido por si usa o no, yo comprendo que él tiene voluntad de usarlo pero no puede."*) The "cannot" is not clear. Nor is it clear what she meant when she said "He can (could) use something [or has the ability to use something], but I can't make a fuss about it because he can't tolerate it" (*"Él poder (podía) usar algo, pero no puedo armarle una escena porque él no lo puede tolerar"*). The last sentence can be interpreted to mean either that the husband cannot stand a fuss or scene over the use of contraceptives or that the actual use bothers him somehow. We are robbed of the context of particulars that might give conviction to one argument or the other. The details of how the husband and wife discussed the issue, and in what contexts, are insufficient; it is clear, however, that these remarks index many particulars that traditional coding procedures only obscure.

We could connect the phrase "can't tolerate it" to the preceding remark about inability to use contraceptives to infer that the husband objects to the use of contraceptives on mechanical or perhaps sensual grounds. There is a problem with the English translation—

> He can (could) use something (or has the ability to use something),
> but I can't make a fuss about it because he can't tolerate it

if we read the translation to imply that the last two "it"s in the sentence refer to the use of contraceptives or simply to contraceptives; yet this rendition can be plausible. Another translation could be the following:

> He could use something (if he wanted to), but I can't raise a fuss
> with him (over the matter) because he can't tolerate scenes of this
> sort (a scene of this sort).

Now the emphasis seems to be placed on the husband's not being able to tolerate scenes or arguments or discussions with his wife; but we still cannot be certain whether the "scenes" are the problem or the question of the use of contraceptives themselves. Returning to the earlier remark by the wife,

> I do not make any problems for him, for whether my husband uses (them) or not, I understand that he has the desire to use it but cannot.

the issue might be how we are to understand the statement "he has the desire to use it but cannot." I did not elaborate on the beginning of this response, "*Salgo corriendo*," in my earlier translation because it did not seem to fit there. This brief utterance might be taken to mean that the woman was referring to her actions after sexual intercourse when she "comes out running," presumably heading for the bathroom for her douche. I tried to make her remarks more meaningful by adding "them" in the phrase "for whether my husband uses *them* or not," to suggest the idea of "uses contraceptives," and I also included "it" in the last part of the sentence to stress the reference to contraceptives. I could have translated the fragment in question as ". . . I know he has the desire to use one but he cannot." However, this translation does not immediately provide a convincing interpretation of "but he cannot." We could easily create a "convincing" interpretation, but this would obscure the issues involved in eliciting information, translating the materials, constructing an interpretation, and recognizing that our everyday expressions are always embedded in more complicated settings, including settings in which the talk itself may be superfluous or misleading.

The foregoing discussion suggests that we might attribute the husband's desire not to use contraceptives to dislike for their "texture" or "feel" or to the time-consuming efforts needed to use them. Or we might assume that there exists some fear of their use that remains implicit, or that he simply does not care to use them because he wants eleven children and his wife only wants three (although we assume him to know that for medical reasons his wife is not to become pregnant again for another year). The substantive content can be manipulated in each analysis by adding or dropping particulars or by stressing some and not others. We can add various particulars to the wife's remarks about seldom talking to her husband about activities they might share, to facilitate the conclusion that this issue is a basic source of familial conflict. Or we might conclude that the sexual encounters are infrequent, and that her remark about 'running out,' presumably after intercourse, is intended to reveal how she tries to avoid further contact with her husband after sexual intercourse. Or we could suggest that all these issues mask more basic problems in the marriage which even a three-hour intensive interview cannot uncover.

The respondent provided information that went beyond the usual answers to fixed-choice questions about conditions that can affect fertility rates. In our interviews we assumed that if the situation was "right"—that is, if the interviewer was convincing in displaying an interest in the respondent's circumstances, or if the respondent used the interview to unburden herself of some thoughts about matters she seldom would discuss with others—then we might acquire considerable information that cannot be coded effectively within the survey analysis. These "right" conditions, which are very difficult to describe, are like trying to give a precise account of one's "warm" or "friendly" feelings toward someone whose acquaintance has been made recently. The "right" conditions are contingent on an emergent and changing interactional setting. Different questions may cause the immediate "warm" relationship to become rather cold, whereas another question accompanied by appropriate glances and voice intonation may cause a respondent to open up.

The subtleties of language use are present in all research but are seldom viewed as integral ingredients in the researcher's claims about "findings." By merely presenting my tables, I could have easily convinced the reader that a relationship between ideal family size and actual family size, as cross-tabulated with church attendance, provides a fairly clear understanding of Argentine fertility. By opening up the issue of how a question is posed by the researcher and how it is interpreted by the respondent, and by asking how in comparative research we are to locate and translate a response and then code it, we uncover social meanings that traditional social research either distorts or fails altogether to handle.

THE HUSBAND'S VIEW. The preceding discussion can be clarified by disclosing some of the remarks made by the husband of the women respondent. The reader should recall that it had been difficult to obtain an interview with the wife—yet the interview with the husband (the night before) had been even more difficult to secure. The wife gave the interviewers various appointments for the husband but the husband never made an appearance. After several such incidents another appointment was made, but this time the interviewers did not show up. The wife complained about this the next time an appointment was requested. On a later occasion the male interviewer encountered the husband at home but could only talk to him through a small screened opening in the door. They arranged for an interview for the coming Sunday at 9:00 A.M. The designated Sunday turned out to be the first of Daylight Saving Time in Buenos Aires, and the interviewer arrived an hour late by the newly instituted schedule. Saying that her husband had waited for an hour and then had left for work, the wife indicated that the husband did not know when another interview could be arranged. On a subsequent afternoon the female interviewer encountered the husband at home during her visit to the wife and was allowed to begin the interview with the husband. After about ten minutes he stopped the interview and said he had to go. The husband indicated that a new appointment could be made, but several more were broken in the ways mentioned previously.

For the next few days the male interviewer returned but did not find the husband at home; each time the wife made the same excuse about having to go to work. At this time the wife was also claiming that she had no time for her interview. She indicated that if someone came by at 4 in the afternoon on any day she would grant an interview, if she were at home. The female interviewer passed by the house two days later at the hour designated but the wife was not home. The husband was there, however, and another appointment was made for his interview the coming Sunday at 9:00 A.M. The male interviewer returned on Sunday but no one answered the doorbell, although a window was open (which usually signified that someone was home). The interviewer went away to check on another family and returned at 9:30 A.M. but again received no answer. While leaving the building he encountered the wife returning from shopping. She said that her husband was still sleeping because he had not retired until 5:00 A.M. and that the interviewer should return at 11:00 A.M. At 11:00 the interview began and lasted for two hours before being terminated by the husband. Another meeting was arranged for the following evening. The husband was not at home at the appointed hour, but the interviewer remained nearby and returned to the house after seeing the husband return some 40 minutes later. He was invited to enter but was told to wait for the interview until the husband had bathed. The interview was finally completed.

The male interviewer obtained informal knowledge of the husband's activities when he encountered the husband on several other occasions, both in the neighborhood and elsewhere (e.g., at Mar del Plata, the popular seaside resort city south of Buenos Aires, where he was losing heavily at the gambling casino).

The interviewers in this case made many comments to me about the difficulties of obtaining the interviews, and they discussed with the respondents the "truthfulness" of various answers. The male interviewer stated that obtaining answers once the interview commenced was not a problem, but that obtaining the initial interview had been difficult because everyone was busy. The wife praised the patience of the interviewers, and the husband said that he had agreed to the interview because he found the interviewer to be a pleasant person. We could speculate that the family—at least the husband—was trying to decide what we were "really" up to and what kind of trust they might reasonably assume. Despite the apparently good relations between the husband and the interviewer, the latter reported that the husband resisted many of the questions on ideal family size and the related questions that followed. This resistance persisted despite many occasions when the two men had drinks together or held long conversations while consuming *máte* (a strong tea drink which is drunk from a gourd passed back and forth between the participants as additional hot water is added).

During one discussion in the presence of both interviewers, the wife returned to the topic of respondents' truthfulness. The male interviewer said that respondents are usually truthful and noted that the husband had frankly confessed to leaving the house on one occasion to avoid seeing the researcher. After the interviews were completed, the male interviewer encountered the husband, who asked how the interview with his wife compared with his own. The interviewer said that he did not know and that the schedule had been turned in. The husband continued to ask about his own case, attempting to ascertain how much personal interest his case held for the interviewer.

From the foregoing remarks, we gather that the relationship of the interviewer to the respondent establishes and reestablishes conditions for asking and answering questions as the interview unfolds. However, if we are preoccupied with obtaining determinate, substantive outcomes (e.g., ideal versus actual family size), we may not recognize that the respondent is making his own judgments about the bits of information he offers— information that is at variance with the researcher's use of traditional fixed-choice questionnaires to seek so-called objective facts that can be coded and summarized in tables.

The husband provided several anecdotes revealing the kind of social activities he pursued—going to dances and bars, drinking, fighting, and engaging in a lot of "horseplay" with his friends. The respondent had only completed primary school, yet had taken over his father's scrap metal business. He also had an interest in singing, particularly tangos. He often went out with "the boys," despite objections by his wife. He noted that he had gambled a lot, once having lost the equivalent of about $3300 at the casino. Presumably the father's business was profitable, for at 28 the respondent owned an automobile and had access to considerable sums of money, although there were few other signs of wealth. The husband reported that he was supporting another child—a boy of 7, who lived with his mother in another part of the city. He claimed to visit the little boy every day.

Asked about doing things with his wife, the husband stated that as a rule they went to the cinema and to restaurants and watched television together, although his father's recent death had caused a temporary halt to such entertainment. However, the wife had stated that they shared virtually no activities—seldom eating together, being alone together infrequently, and never dividing household tasks. The wife stated that she and her husband never talked to each other.

When the husband was asked what he and his wife talk about frequently, he said they spoke about his business, but he added that they talk infrequently and that he was a man of few words. Questioned about whether his wife helped with the business, he replied rather emphatically that she did not participate in anything. The wife said that they discussed their daughter only when a problem arose, but the husband stated that they talked about his child by the other woman, noting that the wife considered the matter to be "vulgar." The idea of another child seemed to bother the wife (if we are to accept the husband's account), but she was not asked to discuss the matter in her interview.

When the husband was asked about other fathers and his evaluation of them as such, he replied that all his friends were bachelors and that he was the only "crazy one." When asked if he knew a good mother he cited the mother of his son but did not mention his present wife. He had begun living with the other woman when he was 18 and she was 23 years old. He claimed that the woman never spoke to him of marriage. One day the woman returned from a trip earlier than expected and found him in bed with the wife of a neighbor. They separated the following day. When the husband was asked about his present relationship with the woman, the interviewer reported that he laughed "maliciously," reminding the interviewer that he visited his son every day and that this included the mother as well. The husband remarked that he had not had sexual relations with his present wife until after they were married; when asked how they got along, he stated "well." When pressed for more information, however, he added that they sometimes argued over his frequent absences and that this "going out" resulted in tension that might persist for 15 days. Asked what the wife said during these periods of tension, the husband replied that he did not know because when she began to talk he would go—that when she became angry there was no point in continuing their conversation as far as he was concerned. (This is an extensive paraphrase on my part of *"No sé, cuando empieza hablar me voy. Ella se enoja y listo."* The Spanish implies more than a routine translation would convey).

The husband's accounts of his past experience with women includes enough details to make his story appear plausible. The story about the first child is also believable. There are no details on the nature of his current contacts with the other woman, but the husband seemed to hint that he was obtaining sexual gratification during his visits to his (former mistress and) 7-year-old son. Although there was no explicit reference to the wife's jealousy (and also nothing in her interview), it is difficult to imagine that the husband's visits to his "other family" would be conducive to closer bonds between the present couple. The husband's remarks about his friends being bachelors and he the only "crazy" one, can be linked to his visits to the other woman and to his frequent nights out with "the boys." He acknowledged the arguments with his wife about his going out with his friends. The husband described his marriage as a kind of "crazy," spontaneous circumstance. He claimed that his wife had spoke of marriage but that he had not. He tried to give the impression that he suddenly had decided to get married and had done so without much thought. The husband stated that he should not have married, that he could not stay home because "the street" dominated him, and that he therefore lamented being married.

The following materials from the interview present a few details about the same couple's sexual unions. I have omitted the Spanish version from the appendix because of translation problems similar to those presented in the discussion of the wife's remarks.

When asked whether he discussed sexual relations with his wife and what his ideas on ideal family size were, the husband reported the following:

3. INTERVIEWER. On some occasion do you talk with your wife about sexual relations? (FA 76 HO 85-31)
   RESPONDENT Never.
   INTERVIEWER. What types of things do you talk about?
   RESPONDENT. I don't talk about it.

The husband's previous reference to the marriage as a sudden, spontane-our affair, and his implicit indication that he was unhappy with marriage, or at least with this marriage, can now be linked to his remark that he never discussed sexual relations with his wife and that he simply did not talk to her about much of anything. Yet he later remarked that he and his wife had talked about how many children each would like. He indicated a preference for 12 children, saying that his wife preferred only one. His wife, however, had previously mentioned that she wanted three children.

4. INTERVIEWER. Do you know any married couples who do not have children? How many? (FA 76 HO 85-33)

RESPONDENT. Yes, four or five cases.

INTERVIEWER. Why don't they have children, what do you make of this?

RESPONDENT. I never ask. But it must be because one of the two cannot.

INTERVIEWER. Let's take married couples that you know with no children, what happened in the case of the first couple that you know of this type? (FA 76 HO 85-33a)

RESPONDENT. They are people known because of my business. But I never ask them. I only suppose it (is like this; that one of them cannot).

INTERVIEWER. Do you know a married couple that has one or two children? How many? (FA 76 HO 85-34)

RESPONDENT. Yes, many.

5. INTERVIEWER. Let's take married couples that you know with only one child; what happened in the case of the first couple that you know of this type (FA 76 HO 85-34a)

RESPONDENT. I don't know for any of the cases. But to have one or two children is very natural. Perhaps they don't have the means (conveniences) (resources).

INTERVIEWER. What kind of resources (means)?

RESPONDENT. Money, home. If I did not have money nor home, I wouldn't have them.

INTERVIEWER. How did you come to know about the case of family X? (FA 76 HO 85-34b)

RESPONDENT. They are acquaintances from the business (They are business acquaintances).

When the interviewer asks questions about why other couples have few or no children, it is easy for the respondent to give an answer that can be coded readily. These questions are misleading because they prod the respondent to speculate about other families in the same way that public opinion polls do. This was not the intention of my study. I used these questions to ensure a replication of previous studies. If the questions were closed or fixed-choice, the issue of whether the respondent has talked to others about why they have few or no children might never arise. When the husband said "to have one or two children is very natural" and then mentioned "means" or "resources," we could claim that this fits traditional findings—namely, that many families supposedly restrict their production because of limited resources and that this is a "natural" view among many groups. The husband's responses are presumably based on what he feels is "obvious" about the way others decide such matters. However, researchers use even more condensed information, aggregated across a sample, to produce general explanations of entire populations, but ignoring the respondents' everyday circumstances. The husband omitted mention of his own everyday circumstances and did not say whether he could afford to have 12 children or whether wanting many children is natural for all people having the resources. We could easily link the husband's remarks about the importance of available resources and what is "natural" to his religious views, thus concluding that traditional studies of fertility behavior are supported by the present investigation.

The interviewer continued to ask questions on family size.

6. INTERVIEWER. In general, who do you think likes a large family, men or women?
   RESPONDENT. The men.
   INTERVIEWER. Why do you think that men like a large family more? (FA 76 HO 85-35)
   RESPONDENT. I say this because I like a large family. There is no (consensus) total opinion (unanimous opinion): it is very diffuse (diverse).
   INTERVIEWER. Why do you think that women like a small family? (FA 76 HO 85-35b)
   RESPONDENT. Because this way they have less work.

The husband's flat statement that men prefer large families was amplified when he was prodded to reveal his own bias; then he suggested that "diffuse" or "diverse" reasons existed for the male viewpoint. He reasoned that women preferred small families because fewer children were less work.

7. INTERVIEWER. What do you think is the best (ideal) size for a family (FA 76 HO 85-36)
   RESPONDENT. Fourteen people; twelve children; nine males and three

females. I like children. Look, I am a bundle of nerves. But children can do whatever they like to me and I do not become nervous. What I like best is to return home and have the twelve jump (all over) me (throw themselves all over me).

INTERVIEWER.   Why didn't you have twelve children? (FA 76 HO 85-36a)

RESPONDENT.   Well . . . you (certainly) ask about very personal things!

INTERVIEWER.   It's just that since you like children so much. . . .

RESPONDENT.   Yes, but these are very personal matters. I didn't have more because no more came.

Our interviews suggest the kinds of relationships that must be developed in the exchange to obtain details about everyday behavior and about social and sexual interaction between spouses. For example, the husband avoided answering the question "Why didn't you have twelve children?" by responding "Well . . . you (certainly) ask about very personal things!" But he added that ". . . no more came." In this exchange we presumed subtle details of meaning about the setting that cannot be reproduced simply by providing a transcript of the interview. We do not have additional details from the interviewer indicating how the respondent appeared (in terms of his facial expressions, tone of voice, and movement of his eyes) ; nor do we know how the interviewer felt about and tried to control his own appearance when posing the probes about not having more children. We also cannot present information suggesting that the interviewer had developed a relationship that permitted or encouraged certain liberties that were not present in other interviews.

The interviewer then asked the husband about the wife's views on family size.

8. INTERVIEWER.   What is the ideal family (size) your wife prefers? (FA 76 HO 85-37)

RESPONDENT.   One child. By now I would have liked at least four or five children (Today, at this time I would prefer at least four or five children).

INTERVIEWER.   How do you know that your wife feels (thinks) this way about this matter? (FA 76 HO 85-37a)

RESPONDENT.   Because we talk about it.

INTERVIEWER.   What does she tell you?

RESPONDENT.   That she is satisfied with having only one.

When the husband responded to the questions about the ideal family size preferred by his wife, he made no connection between his answers to previous queries about his relationship to his former common-law wife or to his disagreements with his wife on various domestic problems. If we were to view the foregoing materials as context-free questions and answers, our coding decisions would generate explicit preferences that would be divorced from the many problems uncovered in the probing questions used.

The interviewer asked the husband about having fewer children than the ideal number desired ("It's just that since you like children so much. . . ."), and the husband responded:

> Yes, but these are very personal things (matters). I didn't have more because no more came.

There was no attempt on the part of the interviewer to challenge this response further. The interviewer *did not* suddenly point an accusing finger at the respondent and say "Is it because you and your wife don't get along, because you are unfaithful to your wife and she is fed up with your cheating, because she doesn't let you get near her?" The tacit conditions governing the interview precluded such questions. In our interviews, however, we did obtain candid remarks about the intimacies of everyday married life, covering several reports of abortions among devout Catholics, confessions of incest, and detailed accounts of marriages that have been "simulated" for more than 25 years to maintain appearances among relatives, friends, and neighbors. None of these occurrences should be surprising to the reader, yet the neglect of such situations in many studies of fertility behavior would lead one to think that perhaps they are irrelevant to an understanding of claims based on aggregated fixed-choice responses about population differentials and change.

It is not easy to disentangle the differing accounts given by the husband and the wife. I have tried to reveal how my retrospective and prospective integration of ethnographic details creates plausible explanations for individual cases that would not be revealed by an aggregated table. A table containing discrepancies between husbands and wives in terms of the number of children desired would not retrieve information about day-to-day relationships between spouses, nor would it help us to determine how these relationships can influence fertility behavior. Do we reason that the husband's "wild" ways (going out with the boys and maintaining a long-standing relationship with a former common-law wife) made it impossible for him to have a "happy" marriage with his present wife? Do we argue that the legal wife may have forced her husband to return to the common-law wife for companionship by a mishandling of their mutual interests? Or, do we conclude that the wife could not satisfy her husband sexually and that the availability of the former companion made the present marriage a kind of ritual? Do we propose that almost daily contact with the little boy made some kind of relationship inevitable with the child's mother? Obviously many more conjectures could be made, but the issue is this—how do we use such additional details to suggest particular types of fertility behavior that would be predictable? The details just alluded to merely point to the poverty of our studies on fertility: we have avoided the difficult study of everyday encounters in the home within which the practical circumstances of cohabitation unfold. Instead, we have seized on convenient glosses that can be easily coded. Hence even the details I have presented are insufficient for drawing explicit conclusions about fertility behavior, much less for arriving at the kinds of conclusions that a survey study furnishes.

Further Details on Sexual Unions. I want to discuss briefly one more couple because their interviews contain additional responses and replies seldom emphasized by surveys. This young couple was interviewed on three separate occasions by the same female interviewer. The interviewer reported that the husband answered the door and almost immediately let her into their impoverished one-room shack. The wife sat nearby on the dirt floor. The crowded circumstances made the interview uncomfortable for all parties, and she felt that many questions were avoided and responses altered or condensed because of this arrangement. The husband seemed very friendly but the wife appeared rather cold. The wife seemed to warm up considerably during her interview, and the interviewer described the two visits (four and six days after the husband's interview) as very friendly. In describing the husband's responses, the interviewer noted that he talked extensively about some things, but when the issue of birth control came up he appeared to be blushing; he lowered his head and shrunk back, as if to withdraw or to hide himself, thus revealing as little of his thoughts as possible. He became so withdrawn during this part of the interview that his responses consisted almost entirely of gestures The wife was considered to be more cooperative; she was so helpful and talkative that the interviewer was hard pressed to record the long, detailed answers that were supplied. The interviewer was quite frustrated in trying to reproduce the details of the conversation because there were many glances, gestures, laughs, smiles, and frowns that seemed to signify much more than could be written down when recording a verbal answer to a question. Frequently the interviewer felt that the respondent did not understand the questions, and several other types of phrasing were resorted to; at times, however, the interviewer felt it was impossible to communicate the intent of the question.

At the time of the interview the wife worked as a servant in a private home. The husband had only reached the fourth year of primary school, and the wife, who had repeated the first grade several times, and then dropped out of school, claiming that there were no places available; but she was quite happy with this outcome, since she did not feel she was very bright.

The wife provided many details about how the couple became married after she had borne a child out of wedlock. They were married at 18, and each claimed that the experience had been his first sexual union. The wife said that she had been dating her present husband (boy friend) steadily, and that one night he had accompanied her to the private home where she worked. The pair found that everyone was away, but rather than wake up someone in the custodian's apartment to gain entrance, the boy friend suggested two rooms in a hotel for the night. At the hotel, so the wife's story went, they were told that only one room was available, with a double bed (*cama matrimonial,* or a bed for a married couple). The boy friend said he would sleep on the floor, but the wife stated they ended up sleeping together. They continued having sexual relations for some time until the young woman became pregnant. Her parents were quite annoyed, and a confrontation with the boy friend was arranged; at that time he agreed to marriage, indicating that he had wanted to be married all along but felt it advisable to wait until the couple had a place to live. The husband had no home of his own available (he said he was not claimed as a legitimate offspring by his father) and did not want to live with the girl's parents.

This was a young Catholic couple who seldom attended church. Both spouses came from low-income families; they lived in a *villa miseria,* had two children, and were expecting the third. The husband said he would like two or three children but claimed not to know what his wife wanted. The wife stated she would like four children and assumed that she would have them. But she pointed out to the interviewer that, with the third child on the way, she would almost have one child for each year they were married. She felt this would be too much and asked how she might control the situation. The wife indicated (as did the husband) that she did not know any methods for not having children, and she asked for advice. The interviewer explained several methods and advised the wife to consult a doctor and to use a diaphragm for maximum security. There appeared to be no discussion between the husband and wife about how many children each wanted or about controlling the number of children they might have. Yet in answering the question about why some couples have only one or two children, the husband answered:

> [A literal translation would begin "Over there one wants. . . ." I will use a free translation, as follows.]
> These people want no more than one or two because of economic reasons in order to raise them well.
> *Por ahi uno quiere tener 1 o 2 no mas por causas economicas para criarlos bien.*

This answer seems to support the findings of those fertility studies which report that many families desire few children because of economic reasons and because they want to give their offspring more advantages in life.

When the husband was asked how many children he would want if he could start all over again, and what the best number for the family of a man in his economic position would be, he replied that he would like the three (counting the pregnancy of the wife at the time) he now had ". . . because it is also not a question of filling yourself up with children." It would appear that, like the wife, he had some concern with controlling the number of children in the family. But both spouses seemed to profess ignorance of contraceptives, and according to their responses they did not discuss the number of children each wanted. When the wife was asked to give the "best" number of children for a family of their economic standing, she replied, ". . . two, because life (living) is expensive. Even those who can have them say this."

The foregoing case seems to be "typical"—a poor family with little education, uninterested in religious activities, living in a one-room shack, and having no knowledge of contraceptives. Opinions expressed by both husband and wife implied that the couple had thought about having fewer children, but they seemed to have done nothing about family planning. There is no reason to deny that married couples of all economic levels probably give some thought to the size of family they want; in their everyday living, however, the issue may never be as concretized as it appears in the interview situation. The questions we asked could have helped to crystallize the recognition that a limit to family size was desired.

Conclusions. The recorded answers of an interview are seldom self-evident to the researcher. The questions asked of a respondent trigger many thoughts that do not represent the theoretical issues we seek to render operational by different questionnaire items. The interview setting generates its own activities, even when that elusive and indescribable delicate balance we call "rapport" is not altered. The varied conditions of interaction leading up to and occurring during the actual interviewing sessions are not reflected in the tables constructed by researchers. I have presented some of the details of the interviews in an attempt to indicate how researchers can normatively organize particulars in constructing convincing accounts about fertility behavior. The tables carry an implicit but inadequate depiction of the ethnographic details used in eliciting and coding information considered to be relevant to fertility studies.

A demographer or population sociologist interested in population problems might be quite impatient with the preceding discussion; he might want to shout out rather emphatically that we cannot assemble "objective" evidence by treating each case in the way I have done here. My procedure would preclude compiling elegant tables summarizing precise "findings"; hence it would make it difficult to propose the "real" causes of fertility differentials. Probing into each question and answer sociolinguistically and ethnographically would mean treating each case as a separate sample. The value of a sample survey would be sharply reduced, except as an expedient way of obtaining quick and condensed substantive findings that could be used for policy issues. The policy decisions would be based on rough approximations but not on convincing findings.

APPENDIX   SPANISH VERSION OF INTERVIEW MATERIALS

1. Q: ¿Habla Ud. alguna vez con su marido (esposa) acerca de relaciones sexuales? (FA 76 MU 163-31)
   A: Si.
   Q: ¿De qué tipo de cosas habla Ud.? (FA 76 MU 163-31a)
   A: Dentro de lo sensual, hablámos que para mi marido, la cama representa el 95% del matrimonio, para mi solo 5% [muchas sonrisas]. Para mí es un complemento, yo no concibo cómo para algunas mujeres todo se arregla en la cama. Para mí si todo lo demás anda mal, si discuto con mi marido, si hay peleas, no puede ser que todo se olvide cuando uno se va a dormir con él. ¿No le parece?
2. Q: ¿Conoce Ud. matrimonios que no tengan hijos? ¿Cuántos? (FA 76 MU 163-33)
   A: Uno.

Q: ¿Por qué no tienen hijos, qué le parece a Ud.? (FA 76 MU
163-33a)

A: Porque él no quería tener.

Q: Tomemos cada familia sin hijos que Ud. concoce: ¿Como se
enteró? (FA 76 MU 163-33b)

A: [No response. Interviewer indicates the last answer satisfies this
question as well.]

Q: ¿Conoce Ud. algun matrimonio que tenga uno o dos hijos?
Cuántas? (FA 76 MU 163-34)

A: 1, una hermana.

Q: Tomemos los matrimonios con un solo hijo que Ud. conoce,
¿qué ocurrío en el caso de la primera pareja que Ud. conoce de
este tipo? (163-34a)

A: Quería uno, después se cuidó y ahora quiere y no puede.

Q: (Para cada familia con uno dos hijos, preguntar:) "¿Cómo
se enteró en el caso de la familia X?" (163-34b)

A: [No response. Interviewer indicates that the last answer was
viewed as satisfying this question.]

Q: En general, ¿a quiénes les gusta más una familia grande, a los
hombres o a las mujeres? (163-35)

A: Tanto uno como otro. [Two probes were to be used here, but
the interviewer does not indicate what happened.]

Q: ¿Cuál cree Ud. que es el mejor tamaño de una familia? (163-36)

A: 3 hijos.

Q: [Si el número dado como el "mejor tamaño" es differente del
numero real de hijos en la familia de la entrevistada/o, preguntar:] "¿Por qué Ud. no tuvo X hijos?" (163-36a)

A: Porque tengo que esperar 1 año y medio después que tuve la
nena. La Doctora me lo recomendó así. Quedé delicada.

Q: ¿Cuál es el tamaño ideal de una familia para su marido? (163-37)

A: 11 hijos.

Q: ¿Cómo sabe que su marido piensa así sobre este asunto? (163-37a)

A: Le encantan los chicos; de soltero ya decía eso.

CHAPTER 9

SOCIOLINGUISTIC FEATURES OF FERTILITY INTERVIEWS

The interview materials reported in previous chapters were obtained from the interviewer's notes, which were taken (usually verbatim) during the exchange between the interviewer and the respondent. When the researcher attempts a textual analysis without a tape-recorded interview, it is difficult to record details not directly elicited by the planned questions; the interviewer becomes preoccupied with writing down information he thinks is relevant to the topics designated by the questionnaire. A tape-recorded version of the interview provides a clearer picture of how the setting generates information that is independent of the stimulus conditions structured by the questionnaire. In this chapter I focus on the complexities of the elicitation procedure and on the recognition of relevant information.

In discussing the interview described below I use both the interviewer's notes and the transcript of the tape recording. The interview was done in Lanus, a working-class suburb of Buenos Aires. The couple interviewed had had a common-law marriage of 17 years' duration. The husband was very difficult to interview despite several attempts made by the interviewer and despite apparent friendliness toward the male interviewer, with whom the husband was most willing to go drinking. The husband drank frequently and often abused his wife by beating her, insulting her verbally, and carrying out activities described only as "foolish" by the interviewer. Evidently the initial meeting was readily arranged and required little explanation of the rationale of the interview. An appointment was made to interview the wife two days later. On the agreed day, however, it was difficult to conduct the interview because the husband was at home and drunk. He monopolized the conversation, made demands on his wife, and prevented the usual exchange of questions and answers.

The husband insisted that the (female) interviewer remain for lunch. Frequent toasts were made, and the husband interrupted many of the toasts with a guitar accompaniment. Quantities of wine were offered to everyone. The wife did not say much during this encounter, although she laughed occasionally and rebuked the husband for his rude talk and ". . . lack of respect for a married woman." The interviewer tried to engage the husband in a dialogue on some of the questions, but the husband, who always avoided giving his opinions, talked about various topics that seemed to emerge as if by free association.

When she accompanied the interviewer to the door, the wife began talking a great deal about her situation with her partner. It was then that she indicated that she was not married to the man but had been living with him for the 17 years. She described his drinking habits and the behavior he exhibited while drunk. The wife connected her remarks about her relationship with this man, and about his drinking, to magical explanations for the individual's behavior. She said that a person in the neighborhood who wanted to take her husband away from her had thrown salt and sugar under the door and that one of the couple's children had stepped on the mixture, thus causing a misfortune to hover over the household. The wife indicated that she believed in spirits, told fortunes by reading cards and palms, and possessed a fountain of knowledge that was infallible. Thus no one could fool her.

The female interviewer expressed her confidence at the outset that the wife would prove to be very cooperative because the latter seemed to be quite interested in the general description of the interview; she seemed to be interested in talking about her own problems, and even seemed to accept the presence of the tape recorder as an indication of the importance of her opinions and ideas. The interviewer came to feel especially optimistic about the responses she was receiving when some neighbors interrupted the interview, whereupon the wife told the visitors that the interview was necessary because it would provide professionals with information about problems people had within their families and in raising children. But the interviewer also felt that the woman might be too cooperative; for example, the respondent seemed inclined to use any question posed as an introduction to a variety of other topics not connected with the questionnaire. Yet the interviewer was reluctant to cut the woman off too soon, perhaps losing valuable information about the everyday life of the family. Finally, the interviewer felt that the respondent, despite her tendency to disgress with each question, seemed to return to a few intense experiences of her life that preoccupied her thinking and her answers throughout the interview.

Unlike the cases described previously, the present interview was conducted in an atmosphere that the interviewer interpreted as open and direct, and it seemed to produce convincing information. I call attention to the interviewer's remarks because they highlight a central issue—namely, the carefully prepared wording of the questionnaire is antithetical to the various ways in which members communicate their experiences to different audiences. Each interview becomes a particular event, and despite the careful wording and presentation of the questionnaire, the interview generates a highly variable collection of conditions and different kinds of information, which are subject to variable interpretation. The variable interpretation of the interview conditions and information cannot be resolved by standardized coding procedures.

To provide some continuity with previous quotations from other interviews, I discuss the same questions about sexual relations and their relationship to the number of desired offspring versus the actual number of children. The subject tape was originally transcribed by the interviewer, and I found that she had omitted many details from the recorded dialogue. Some of the missing details typify a kind of glossing that occurs when "preparing" data for analysis; but other features are important because they include subtleties seldom covered by a survey-oriented researcher. Hereafter, italic type indicates the interviewer's spontaneous interpolation to the standardized question in Spanish; brackets indicate my own comments. The Spanish version forms an appendix at the end of the chapter. In the English translation of responses and questions, material in parentheses represents alternate possible meanings (as employed in previous chapters), and my remarks about the translation or the interaction implied appear in brackets. At times the interviewer or the respondent breaks into the other's remarks. When the interruption is brief, the comment is merely inserted between slashes. We begin with the section of the schedule that asks about early knowledge of sexual relations.

1. INTERVIEWER. What do you think a young person ought to know about sexual relations (*do you understand me?*) before starting to go out with a man? (FA 115 MU 195-28) (What sorts of things should a young gal know, right?, when she starts to [pause] before going out with a young man, about this problem, about (or on) this problem of sexual relation? [Question repeated and changed.]

RESPONDENT.   Uh, can this mean me? (that this can mean me?) [Not in original transcription.]

INTERVIEWER.   Right (I see, of course), according to your experience, okay? [Notice that the Spanish indicates a shift to the familiar form of speech.]

RESPONDENT.   I would go out with this, this distrust (mistrust, suspicion), okay?

INTERVIEWER.   Aha. Thinki. . . . [Changes her remarks before completing the word.] Yes but, but why mistrust, uh?

RESPONDENT.   Because one does not really know a person (because really one does not know a person that well; because one really does not know a person), because one only knows him like this (casually or superficially) and that's it (because you just know him sort of and nothing more). [You know him but really don't know anything about him.] One has to know herself [him?] deeply (well, in depth) until that moment comes to us (know oneself in depth when that moment comes to us) /INTERVIEWER: right (of course) / or what intentions are there (what intentions are involved.) [The way in which the respondent was attempting to reference herself as opposed to some hypothetical man is not clear because in Spanish she seemed to move from a distrust of men to a concern with one's ability to deal with men under unspecified conditions.]

In the section of the interview preceding the dialogue just given, the respondent discussed her prior relationships with men. She told in detail of her previous common-law marriage, which had resulted in children who were subsequently taken away from her by their father. The descriptions of this earlier alliance included many comments about how men could not be trusted and these attitudes seem to carry over in the present discussion. Although the present husband was described as "better" than the first (who, we were told, was a professional thief), the woman did not fail to mention the present husband's drinking problem. Rather than referring to these previous parts of the session, however, the interviewer probed the use of the term "distrust."

The wife's response to the probe about distrust is of interest because it can be read as autobiographical and as pointing to times of enormous troubles (partially described earlier in the interview). We must ask how we are to interpret and pinpoint particular answers to questions of this sort. It is obviously possible for the respondent to furnish a pat answer by endorsing one alternative of a precoded, fixed-choice question, or by simply saying "men are not to be trusted." The researcher never knows exactly how much biographical material about the respondent will be needed to interpret such answers.

The respondent's elaboration of what she meant by her distrust of men cannot be divorced from her experiences in two common-law marriages. Among other things, she had said that she felt her first husband was sexually abnormal because he demanded a great deal of sex and also because he possessed what she described as an unusually large penis (whose dimensions were indexed by continual reference to a broom that was nearby). The respondent stated that all the first husband did to her was to fill her with babies, and whenever he touched her (inside or outside her body) he smashed or burst her insides. She blamed him for gynecological troubles she experienced. When she talked of her first husband's insatiable sexual appetites and his sexual relations with her, she used the word "animal." It is easy to interpret the respondent's references to the necessity of "really" knowing a person well before submitting sexually, as indexing her past misfortunes with men. Perhaps, on the other hand, the respondent was attempting to indicate that being forced to think about a person whom she felt she knew had made her experiences assume a very conditional quality, and that she was deliberately confronting the problems of sustaining her thoughts about this person in the face of an interview that created a "moment of truth," which seemed to foster new conceptions or to change previous conceptions radically. A constant problem in the interview being described was remaining aware that the respondent was sustaining accounts that might have been idealized versions of what life had been or was presently like, in the face of memories evoked by the interview (memories of experiences that contrasted radically with the idealized accounting schemes).

The interviewer continued with questions about sexual relations with men before marriage.

2. INTERVIEWER. Now, about the concrete problem, about the problem of what a young gal ought to know about sexual relations before starting to go out with young men? [The interviewer paraphrased the original question again.]

RESPONDENT. Well [pause] the problem that they would (ought to) have is of, of knowing what intentions this person has.

INTERVIEWER. [repeating the respondent's last five words] What intentions this person has. Now the young gals with whom you were brought up (you grew up with and/or went around with), how did they learn about the problem of sexual relations between man and woman? (FA 115 MU 195-28a) [The question is slightly changed by adding "now" and substituting "with whom" in place of simply "the young gals or girls you grew up with." Also the plural of man and woman was used

	in the questionnaire.] (Do you remember? How did you yourself learn about it?)
RESPONDENT.	Let me tell you that (I should tell you that) I had few, few friends, I had few girlfriends. /INTERVIEWER: *Aha.*/ If I had them, I had them only recently. ["If I have had any friends," she seems to be saying, "it has only been of late that I have had them."] Every type of person comes to see me that asks me for an explanation, if I can give it to her, I give it to her, if not, I don't give it to her because I don't know what /INTERVIEWER: *Of course, right*/ this [sic] (can) have (contain), okay? But I am a person that is not friendly about having friends (I am the kind of person who is not taken to having friends). Nor making visits of any type to any place (nor do I just make any kind of visit or just to any place).
INTERVIEWER.	Then how did you come to learn about this problem? [The original question was: "How did you come to be informed?"] (FA 115 MU 195-28b) [Cut off by respondent.]
RESPONDENT.	By means of listening to the, the landladies [women she worked for as a servant] that talked (talking), or they would advise me, this is advisable (will suit you), the other guy doesn't suit you. [pause] Thus, my having children, they would say this man is not suitable for you because of this or that, the little money that you have he will take from you (or go off with).

The respondent answered the questions about what the young girls she grew up with knew about sexual relations by referring to the nature of a man's intentions, and then by noting that in any event she had had few at that age. These remarks about a lack of friends may be tied to the earlier question about what a young person ought to know about sexual relations—when the respondent had asked if she could answer for herself, she might have been hinting that she did not know many other girls, nor did she know how they learned about sexual relations. We could also stretch this point to include her subsequent remarks about men and about the importance of "knowing" them well, yet the respondent seemed to be suggesting that it was difficult to know anyone well. We could go one step further by proposing that all questions seemed to touch on the woman's miserable (by her account) existence at the hands of two difficult men. The questions and some of the answers seemed to provide occasions for telling her story to the interviewer, and apparently our questions were well suited for eliciting one episode after another. The respondent's remarks about learning about sexual matters and about men in general from the women who employed her as a servant, suggest that she had stumbled through different experiences. For example, knowing a man who was very demanding sexually made it difficult for her to care for the couple's children, especially since he (being a professional thief) was only home long enough to "burst" her insides from sexual intercourse and leave her pregnant, and since he simultaneously kept other women. Then she reported meeting another man whose wife had been treating him like her first husband had treated her. But meeting the second man in her life, which she described as happening quite by accident, seemed to be a fortuitous experience for her now, in the light of the 17 years they had lived together.

These materials illustrate a few points leading up to the questions about sexual relations with the husband and about the number of children desired. The interviewer did not always read each question as it was written on the questionnaire, and she sometimes repeated herself or altered the question. This practice is customary in all interviewing, despite careful training given interviewers. The context of the interview makes it difficult for the interviewer to follow the exact wording, and it is quite tedious to record all the changes one makes. The dialogue discusses a setting that is displaced by the talk of the present interview. The original setting was unavailable to the participants, and the questions from the schedule imposed an abstract context. From listening to the tape, I gathered that the interviewer was continually straining to direct the respondent's attention to the formal questions. The interviewer's voice seemed to take on a slight edge at times, suggesting that she was trying to push the respondent but did not want to inhibit spontaneous remarks that might be interesting. My observations are similar to those described at length by the interviewer in her written account of the interview.

The interviewer evidently was altering the questions even as she expressed them, presumably because the standard format seemed to be inadequate for the occasion. All interviewers encounter this problem, and depending on the rigidity of their instructions or on their involvement in the task of interpreting the setting, they may simply repeat a question several times, then proceed to the next. Or an individual may change the wording in midquestion, or rephrase the question after having read it according to the schedule. In my own interviewing, I have always tried to put into context such factors as the respondent's face, his past remarks to similar questions, and his difficulty with the language of the questionnaire. Then I try to alter my presentation, either to soften the impact of a question that might embarrass the respondent or to make an item more meaningful to the respondent. The same thing was done when the question about any female's prior knowledge of sexual relations was immediately turned into a question about the respondent, and the interviewer encouraged this interpretation. This is a common occurrence. The respondent may not feel confident about interpreting how others know something or what they think. On the other hand, middle-income respondents may prefer a third-party vehicle for expressing views about themselves.

Traditional survey questionnaires seek answers that will reveal patterns presupposed by the formulation of the items themselves. Many low-income respondents receive and process questions against a background of experiences that they cannot articulate sufficiently well to provide the kind of normative accounts researchers hope for and they try to elicit with questionnaire items. Researchers have virtually no knowledge of how many members of a population sampled are more practiced than others in generating "convincing" accounts. All researchers must construct their guesses about what respondents think of their questions and their intentions; they must decide how much credence to place in the respondents' actual answers to researchers' questions. Researchers are forced to scrutinize their methods for generating research accounts, just as they are forced to examine the way in which respondents produce accounts for themselves and researchers.

Attitudes About Sexual Relations. Continuing with the questions asked of the same female respondent, I turn to a section that revealed more about her sexual relationships with her husbands than was learned from later questions, which were designed to trigger discussions on this topic. As indicated in earlier chapters, many questions were asked to maximize the possibilities of obtaining information about a particular issue. Particular questions at specific occasions in the interview did not elicit the information desired, whereas other questions, perhaps more tangential, generated many details sought in a previous question. This type of questionnaire (see example below) is necessary if one takes seriously the differential rapport and changing relationship between interviewer and respondent.

3. INTERVIEWER. Now with what frequency (Now how often) do you think that a person needs to have (it is necessary for a person to have) [sexual] relations? [The question should have been:

"How often do you think a person needs to have sexual relations in order to be happy." (FA 115 MU 195-28i)] [The prior discussion was about sexual relations and I am assuming that this was obvious to both respondent and interviewer. The answer certainly implies this interpretation.]

RESPONDENT.   Uh, according to one's natural desires (what comes naturally).

INTERVIEWER.   Now, right, now how often, if we take one week as a base, for example, or a month, how many times a month do you think, for example, does a person need to have sexual relations to live normally, in other words. Take a week for a basis [for your answer], what do you think is better than a month? And how many times a week? [mumble trailing off.]

RESPONDENT.   Do you mean have sex? [This is my free interpretation of the intention of the response. I could not hear the tape clearly and followed the interviewer's transcription.]

INTERVIEWER.   Yes, yes, yes. [not in transcription]

RESPONDENT.   Uh, it depends, it could be every day, or it could be every three days, every four days.

INTERVIEWER.   Right. It depends on the person, you say.

RESPONDENT.   Of course [The respondent cut herself off before completing the utterance.] It could be, and also one cannot say.

INTERVIEWER.   Right, right. I was talking about (referring to) women that would sometimes tell me [pause] give me (tell me) a high frequency, you see, they would give me [cut off by respondent].

By asking how often one "needs" to have sexual relations, the interviewer presupposes that a respondent has given some thought to the matter. The question is quite open ended and we assume that respondents will base their answers on their personal desires. In this case the respondent made a very general answer, and the interviewer began to push for a more specific opinion by asking the respondent to use a week as a basis for her answer, then a month, and then again a week, finally asking how many times during the week. Apparently the interviewer (who simply let her voice trail off) did not quite know how to handle the question or how to phrase the reference in terms of a period of time. In a number of places (e.g., at the words *"en fin"*—"in other words"), it appeared that the interviewer was trying to encourage an answer without having to release more details about her interest in asking the question. The response was also inexplicit when the respondent used the term *"uso"* ("use" or "activity"), but I assumed that both interviewer and respondent were referring to sexual relations. The respondent finally remarked that the desirable frequency of sexual relations "depends."

We could interpret this ambiguity to mean that the respondent was simply not clear in her own mind, perhaps because she had not thought about it much, or that she was embarrassed to reveal her views. The interviewer said "right" and repeated the respondent's remarks, presumably waiting for further detail. The respondent began by saying "*logic(o)*" or "of course," as if it were all clear; then she started to say more but finished by saying ". . . also one cannot say." It appeared that the respondent could not give a specific answer to such a general question.

The interviewer's last remark in this sequence (see below) was "right, right." She then switched her tactics, assuming that the respondent intended to repeat her own exaggerated notions of the frequency of sexual activities of other women. When the respondent cut off the interviewer, it was not clear whether she now comprehended the earlier line of questioning and the "hints" and was willing to be more direct in her reply, or whether the respondent's reference to her husband signaled a way she *could* answer a question otherwise perceived as being too general.

4. RESPONDENT.   Take my husband, the way he is, with his age, (There you have my husband as you can see him, at his age) if it were up to him, it would be every night. I get tired (of it. It tires me out.)

INTERVIEWER.   Right, right. [Not in transcript.]

RESPONDENT.   Now the other [first husband] no [is not like this, presumably because he was seldom home], the other would . . . would miss six months, three months and [pause—Inaudible low voice trailing off for about three words. Then both began to speak simultaneously.] . . . if it was every night, young lady, every night, uh it just couldn't be.

INTERVIEWER.   As he (you) came [home] tired ["the other husband," or "as you came home tired?"—and the voice trails off].

RESPONDENT.   [Cutting off the interviewer:] It doesn't interest him (if I am tired.) [This would mean that she was not referring to her first husband, but the second, the one who would like sex every night. This means that the interviewer's remarks ("as he comes home tired") would have to mean as "one comes home tired."] So, he still says even when I satisfy him that I don't have [everything in it] something over there and that can't be. [This is not clear to me. I think she is saying that although she accommodates him sexually, he acts as if it is not enough on her part.] If one's own age does not permit it. Every three days, every four, every six, and every week is the most [one can imagine.] [It is difficult to indicate where sentences begin and end in listening to the tape. I cannot perceive obvious pauses that would suggest clear sentence boundaries.]

The interviewer's reference to the high frequency of sexual activity reported by other women as described earlier was followed by a direct reference to the respondent's present husband, this establishing the intent of the earlier question—to find out about the respondent's and husband's views concerning frequency of sexual relations. The respondent's reference to her husband's age semed to imply that even "with his age" or despite his age, he would like sexual relations every night. The interviewer's *"right, right"* implied agreement that every night is too much. The respondent's reference to the other husband terminates with both women speaking simultaneously and the respondent returning to her view that every night was too much. We still do not know precisely what the respondent considered to be an "adequate" frequency for having sexual relations; but we have learned that the present husband wanted sex too often, whereas the former husband, who was often absent for long periods, was described as like an "animal" when he was home.

The interviewer's next remark about coming home tired is not clear, since we are not sure whether it was the husband or the wife who came home tired. Thus if we assume the present husband was being discussed, it may (or may not) be that the respondent came home tired but tried to satisfy her husband, only to find that her actions were not appreciated. Neither the Spanish version nor my translation is very clear here. Perhaps the woman was saying that her present husband was not satisfied with her efforts to please him sexually, but her age did not permit a more vigorous attempt. She then seemed to commit herself to the statement that sexual relations every three to seven days was all she could manage.

5. INTERVIEWER. This is a. . . . [I cannot decipher the last two words.]
   RESPONDENT. Yes. I say it because [pause] one's age, in other words [in short] . . . [both are now talking at once and a few words are lost] Now you are still a younger gal /INTERVIEWER: *right/* a lady that, in other words that still [already], right?
   INTERVIEWER. Yes, yes, yes. Well, and so everything, also, the [pause] it can't be this way every night, right? It just can't be. [The respondent breaks in almost simultaneously as the interviewer produces these last three words, and for a few moments they both talk at the same time.]
   RESPONDENT. No, no, it can't be, but [pause] the doctor has told him, the same doctor [then two inaudible words] has told him that he

is very strong [he has a lot of stamina] /Interviewer breaks in
with "right, right"/ by nature [has a strong constitution].
INTERVIEWER: of course, of course. /He eats well! He drinks
well! [voice rising and emphatic]

INTERVIEWER. In other words he is always more than ready.

Numerous possible meaning-structures are lost in the course of this
broken and not entirely reproducible dialogue. Yet the disjointed interchanges ("now you are a younger gal /Inter. *"right"*/, a lady that, in other
words still [already], right?") could be taken to imply that each "knew"
what the other was saying. Facial and body movements that would contribute to our understanding of the dialogue cannot be captured by hear-
ing the tape, yet when I listen to the tape I have the feeling that each
participant wanted to convey the impression that she was clear about the
other's intentions. I can easily assume that the wife was noting that the
interviewer, as a younger woman, might not feel the age problem in
having sexual relations with her husband ("a lady that, in other words
still [capable of having frequent sexual relations]"). The interviewer
floundered a little and then repeated that "it can't be this way every
night." The respondent, too, repeated this and again referred to her
doctor's remarks about her husband's virility, observing that the husband
eats and drinks heartily. The interviewer followed with the remark that
the husband "is always more than ready" for sexual relations.

The interview continued with additional questions regarding sexual
relations.

6. INTERVIEWER. [The next question should have been: "Do you ever talk to
your husband about sexual relations?" But this question was
preceded by other talk about how faithful men and women
are to each other and the interviewer seemed to be concerned
with reminding the respondent of the previous discussion about
sexual relations that came inadvertently in questions quoted
earlier. The interviewer asked:] Now, uh, . . . [The next
three words are not clear and the interviewer seemed to be
having trouble deciding how to formulate the question.] Now
I am going to ask if you talk like this, sometime with your
husband [pause], do you remember those problems that we
talked about yesterday? About [pause], the frequency (how
often), how many times you had sex [had occasion to engage
in (sexual) practices] [pause], of these problems that we
spoke of yesterday. Do you talk to him about them? (FA 195
MU 115-31)

RESPONDENT. Yes.

INTERVIEWER. What, about what sorts of things, for example, do you talk to him? (FA 195 MU 115-31a)

RESPONDENT. Are you talking to me about this marriage? [This is not clear. I think I hear "this marriage" but the interviewer did not transcribe the utterance. The tape is difficult to follow here.]

INTERVIEWER. Uh, yes. And what do you tell him about this, or he to you about this?

RESPONDENT. What he tells me is that [pause] that this is the road (the way it is) for a person (someone).

The prior discussion had concerned sexual relations, and it had emerged from questions about the frequency of sex and its presumed importance for one's health. The next question (number 6) sought to approach the problem a little more directly by soliciting information about discussions between the husband and wife. The interviewing involved asking questions that overlapped to ensure that certain topics would be covered. The interviewer reminded the respondent of their conversation of the day before, mentioning the frequency of sexual contact and "those problems that we talked about yesterday." The interviewer employed the term *"uso"* (*"use"*—use, practice, wear, and habit are a few dictionary translations) rather than a term that could be directly translated as "sexual intercourse," thus indexing the topic in an implicit way by borrowing a term the respondent had used earlier apropos of the frequency of sexual intercourse. The interviewer presumed that the context was clear and that, earlier, *"uso"* could only have meant "sexual relations." The interviewer thus built the term *"uso"* into further questioning, even though she had not clarified its meaning earlier.

The respondent's "Yes" to the question about whether she talked to her husband about the frequency of sexual relations, forced the interviewer to probe with "What, about what sorts of things, for example, did you talk to him about?" The tape is difficult to understand here, but apparently the respondent said "Are you talking to me about this marriage?"—"this" presumably designating her present marriage. The visual display available to the interviewer could have suggested the first marriage, but the dialogue does not reveal such particulars. The follow-up by the interviewer pushed the issue again, but the response would certainly not be very helpful to a researcher: "What he tells me is that [pause] that this is the road (the way it is) for a person (someone)." It was necessary for the interviewer to change the reel of tape at this point, and her subsequent questioning did not pursue the topic further. The respondent did not clarify how she talked to her husband about sexual relations, even when she was asked a more direct question (e.g., FA 195 MU 115-31 and the probe—31a). We might infer, however, that the husband received what he demanded and that the woman was resigned to her fate. Perhaps "What he tells me is that [pause] that this is the road (the way it is) for a person (someone) " might also be understood as "That's the way it is going to be," or "That's the way the ball bounces."

Interpreting the tape is very difficult, for there is a normative expectation that I will create sentences that are understandable to the reader, yet I am not at all sure how the material is to be punctuated. I can detect "pauses," but they do not seem to occur in "obvious" places. Once I commit myself to a form of punctuation, however, I also force my materials into particular categories by the way I use English syntax. There is nothing inherently "natural" about the way I might hear pauses, hesitations, or shifts of topics. I am creating pauses, hesitations, and topics by the cultural way I present the materials to the reader. My analysis is structured at the outset by the way I record the questions and the answers orthographically. It is difficult to interpret occasions on which interviewer and respondent talk simultaneously. It may be that their relative intentions or thoughts follow different lines, which sometimes appear to overlap because of their use of vocabulary that is ostensibly the "same." Or, some readers might want to argue that they talk simultaneously because they are thinking of the same thing. The rambling indulged in by both interviewer and respondent is not simply a result of "bad" interviewing, as some readers might want to claim; rather, it is an attempt on the part of the interviewer to encourage and gently urge the respondent into making more spontaneous remarks about her experiences and views. The respondent's digressions suggest that some thought has been given to the matter; but there also seems to be a vagueness that may be integral to the talk or to the original experience. The respondent's categories are no more precise than those used by the interviewer. The language seems to be recognized by the participants as imprecise, yet perhaps adequate for the practical task of the interview.

It is difficult to be clear about how the frequency of sexual relations desired or tolerated by either marital partner might affect the number of offspring the couple could have. Clearly it is hard to ask about the issue of sexual relations desired or tolerated; it is difficult for the respondent to formulate answers. A better-educated respondent might be less bothered because her more formal use of language could enable her to give us categories which—although we might judge them to be difficult to probe or make problematic—we would be required to accept as "data," albeit of dubious validity. An answer of "Several times a week, depending on how we feel" would not reveal how each partner conceived of sexual relations in their marriage, nor how these conceptions can or do influence fertility patterns. This type of answer could be probed, but it would require tactful interviewing, characterized by sensitivity to the respondent's voice intonation and to additional indications concerning the mood of the respondent. A fixed-choice question might provide the respondent the option of "several times a week." Such a response permits the individual to avoid details about problems associated with sexual relations.

The foregoing material is amenable to further breakdowns and interpretations, but let us now terminate the discussion and attend to other issues.

Emergent Sociolinguistic Features in a Textual Analysis of Family Size. The taped dialogue reveals more details than might be evident from handwritten transcriptions alone (e.g., a few indications are given about the apparent mood of the participants and the disjointed character of some of the dialogue). Notice that the transcription does not convey subtleties of intonation, phonetic contrasts, and suggestions of differential enthusiasm on the part of the participants to different portions of the exchange. Equally important, I omitted the details regarding the natives' use of language on which I based my translation and attributed meanings to written segments. When interruptions occurred, I had to look ahead to decide what a fragment might mean, for the word order differences between English and Spanish complicate the translation of fragmentary utterances. Had I attempted to code each questionnaire while listening to a tape of the interview, I would have had to take into account innumerable particulars which would be buried or ignored or suppressed if I were to use supposedly verbatim notes from a written documentation of the interview, simply coding each item as if it were a paraphrased, edited, and presumably independent event.

Moreover, the intonational features of the talk and the knowledge I presume about the way Argentines convey irony, surprise, humor, and so on, cannot be revealed by treating each item, probe, and answer of a tape-recorded interview within the format of a standardized coding procedure. My own views about the way Argentines think, express themselves under different circumstances, mask thoughts, exaggerate, and understate, are essential elements of my coding activities and of my analysis of the translated transcript. By throwing out such information we make our coding practices simple and our data simple-minded. As I try to reflect the ways in which Argentines encode expressions in norma- tively acceptable utterances, I also wish to indicate to an English-speaking audience (perhaps only American English) expressions that reflect typical, "clear" reasoning, or normative structures. Since my thoughts in Spanish (Argentine Spanish) and in English (American English) incor- porate normative syntactic and lexical structures, my translations will be intelligible to American English readers. The demands of sociological research reports, which usually result in the omission of sociolinguistic details, make it difficult for me to describe the organization of my own thinking and the constraints imposed on it by the verbal expressions I am both accustomed to using and expected to formulate for the American English reader. Different interpretations of the "same" materials are inevitable, yet traditional sociological analysis demands some kind of unified conclusion or integration. But the translations are not simply a matter of moving from Spanish to English (or Argentine Spanish to American English), for the problem exists even within American English dialects or English dialects. Thus we cannot speak of the "same" ma- terials in the two languages, since the English version is *created* by the way I transcribe and translate.

There is a break in the dialogue now, since I want to present only the materials relevant to discussions in earlier chapters about desired number of offspring. I have skipped a question about conversations with one's children about sexual problems—the reply was simply "no, no," and the interviewer did not attempt to probe this response.

7. INTERVIEWER. Marriages (couples) that don't have children, do you know (any) ma'am? [There is a pause here and the respondent begins to say something but is cut off by the interviewer with:] Apart from what (the one) you told me (about) recently, do you remember that one gal, apart [respondent again tries to say something but is cut off by the interviewer] . . . apart from her (that one) do you know of another couple that have no children? /Resp.: Yes, of course./ Why don't they have any, how does it strike you (that they have no children)? [The question should have been: "Do you know any marriages (couples) that do not have children?" (FA 195 MU 115-33)]

RESPONDENT. Uh they don't have any because (someone) is, the wife is sick or the man (husband) is sick.

In seeking explicit information about couples with no children, the interviewer reminded the respondent of a previous discussion in which this topic had emerged spontaneously. The researcher's use of the category "marriages with no children" was presented to the respondent as though it were a "natural" usage for her. The researcher presumed that this category would index the "same" conditions for all respondents. The respondent's answer that couples do not have children because one or the other spouse was ill seemed to be a believable one.

The respondent seemed to be searching for ways in which to provide the interviewer with "acceptable" answers—that is, to say whatever she could get away with for the moment or whatever seemed to satisfy the interviewer. The respondent often asked the interviewer for her opinion, or more important, made a kind of response and then inquired whether the answer did not strike the interviewer as "reasonable." The interviewer was forced into a tacit kind of support for the responses, but we cannot be certain whether the respondent was relying on this tacit support in deciding that the answers she was generating were "acceptable."

The questioning now shifts to couples that may have one or two children.

8. INTERVIEWER. Ah, that's why they don't have any. [Not transcribed by interviewer.] Now, what about couples (like this) that have one or two children, do you know any? /RESPONDENT: Yes, I know some./ Now why don't they have more than one, for example?

RESPONDENT. Uh, because of how life is so expensive (living is so expensive), also one doesn't want to load up with children. Because if they buy a kilo of bread, how much is a kilo of bread (these days, today), young lady? [if] they buy a liter of milk, if they are two (if there are two of them) why are (should) they going to load themselves up with one (child) today (now), another tomorrow, another after (tomorrow), and what (can) are these people to do?

INTERVIEWER. *Right, right, right, right.* [voice trailing off]

RESPONDENT. These innocents (poor fools) have to live with handicaps.

INTERVIEWER. Thus they have one and stop (they will have one and then stop?)

RESPONDENT. Uhhhhh of course, I would do the same thing. If I had two (me with two) even if they didn't come [the tape is not clear here] I would want them.

Here the respondent began to mention instances researchers would be happy to hear about, for they included such particulars as the cost of living, the price of bread and milk, and the general observation that such couples would not or do not want to "load up" with children under such circumstances. The respondent's vocabulary seems to be consistent with the kinds of responses obtained in countless other surveys on fertility. But is such "acceptable" talk really credible when this respondent (and others like her) also had many children, did nothing to prevent them, or perhaps talked differently when with others? The traditional procedure is to examine the respondents' knowledge of contraceptives and their ability to procure these within the constraints of their income and education; alternatively, it is argued that religious beliefs or "values" prevent the respondents from exercising a consistent course of action.

The dialogue was not easy to interpret when both interviewer and respondent tacitly assumed meanings that were not clearly indexed by the formal and informal questions and answers provided by the interview. The respondent seemed to be suggesting that couples restricted their fertility for economic reasons. The argument seemed to be that certain (unspecified) couples restricted their output or faced debilitation or hardship from having too many children. The day-to-day circumstances were never discussed, nor were the respondent's own difficulties mentioned, although she herself had had many children. The interviewer seemed to say "right" or "of course" to a response as though she "understood" just what was intended by the speaker. The interviewer then formulated a more succinct "response" by saying "Thus they have one and stop (they will have one and then stop)?" The respondent's comment was slow in coming and sounds more confident when she said "Uhhhhh, of course, I would do the same thing." The exchange has little or nothing to do with the woman's life circumstances, except retrospectively, as if she saw her own condition as negative in light of the questions. Yet the exchange revolved around the kinds of questions supplied by the interviewer. There is no way of knowing from our data whether the woman (or other respondents) had ever given any thought to such matters during their years of fertility. *We should not confuse retrospective talk generated by our instruments with day-to-day experiences.*

The dialogue continues with the standard question about who likes a large family more—men or women.

9. INTERVIEWER. Of course. Now in general, what do you think [she cut off herself here] who likes a large family more, men or women? A family with a lot of kids, who is it that likes it most?
 RESPONDENT. Uh, if they get along well in marriage I think that they both

(the man as much as the woman), it's, it's something that [pause] it's nice isn't it? /INTERVIEWER: Right./ It really is nice, because it's nice to see [pause] a table (with, where there are), say 10, 12 kids, like we were with (when we had) 17.

INTERVIEWER. That's (really) nice, huh?

RESPONDENT. It's nice. In the house oooof [the last word was drawn out like a pause] also my husband's (house) [a garbled word] in Tucumán, how many did they also have (there)? It was a table that, my God! Right? (It was some table, right?)

In this somewhat ambiguous response, there is an implied satisfaction with the respondent's own house when there were 17 children. Whether these are childhood memories of settings that might have been reported as miserable by her own mother cannot be subjected to further speculation from present materials. The tone of voice changed here to suggest nostalgia on the part of the respondent, as if the question stimulated a different train of thought, unrelated to that intended by the interviewer. The respondent did not seem to recognize that her remark about how nice a large family is was inconsistent with her earlier comments about having too many children in an expensive world.

The rural Tucumán area, the respondent's native region, is especially poor. Whose conception of "nice" are we being asked to imagine when the respondent uses that word to refer to her early home existence? I have referred to materials that cut across clock-time and experienced-time to illustrate how difficult it is to interpret survey data when the circumstances of the interview and the recall of past events are not made integral features of the analysis, hence of the production of constructed substantive accounts.

The respondent's apparent nostalgia over having been raised in a large family, her remarks about how the high cost of living made it difficult to have more than one or two children, and her own failure to stop with a few children or try to limit her family—all these factors could be coded and accepted independently as relevant data without implying contradictions.

10. INTERVIEWER. Your parents [the tape become unintelligible for a few words] to see these things. [At this point the respondent cut in and the two spoke simultaneously until the interviewer gave way.]

RESPONDENT. . . . then come the big ones (older ones) and then there are the parents, the grandparents, the great-grandparents, the grandchildren, it's, it's only one [cut off by the interviewer].

INTERVIEWER. It is a very, very large family. /RESPONDENT, eh?/ family . . . !
[Both begin speaking simultaneously and it is difficult to disentangle their remarks.]

RESPONDENT. . . . but for [pause] a mother, to me it's (it seems), a father this is something great in (one's) life, /INTERVIEWER: *right.*/ to see this harmony [the next utterance was said simultaneously with the interviewer cutting in with "Now for you . . ."], who knows?

When the respondent described how nice a large family was when they all sat down to the supper table, the interviewer echoed with "That's (really) nice, huh?" As the respondent seemed to continue this train of thought about the home of her parents and that of [one of?] her husband's, the researcher interjected some remarks that were difficult to transcribe because of the noise on the tape; apparently, she had questioned how "nice" this could have been for the parents. The disjointed conversation seemed to indicate that two persons were talking past each other, despite the apparent similarity of vocabulary that would suggest a common topic of discourse. The respondent's nostalgia continued (invoking the parents, grandparents, great-grandparents, the grand children, etc.), but this attitude seemed to change as the dialogue progressed.

11. INTERVIEWER. For you now, therefore, what do you think is the best size for a family? (FA 195 MU 115-36) [Actual question: "What do you think is the best family size?"] That is, how many children [pause] would you have to have?

RESPONDENT Uh I, I tell you frankly [not too clear, but the respondent seems to be laughing slightly as if to convey the impression she is hesitant because of revealing a kind of minor confession], I would be satisfied with what I (now) have and nothing more.

INTERVIEWER. Nothing more than this, right? [Not transcribed by interviewer.]

RESPONDENT. Nothing, nothing.

INTERVIEWER. Now [the interviewer seems to be laughing—I cannot tell whether in response to the solemn way in which the respondent said "nothing, nothing" or whether perhaps she was embarrassed by the next question], why is it that you did not have two rather than having (have), [slight pause] how many did you have? uhhhh, there are five [they both said "five" simultaneously] no seven [they both said "seven" at the same time].

RESPONDENT. Seven, seven, yes (right, well), but the rest are dead.

INTERVIEWER. Of course, of course, of course. [pause] Why is it then that you did not have [laughing slightly again] no more than two?

RESPONDENT. Because doesn't, because it doesn't [laughing also], how can I tell you (how can I make it clear to you) [all the foregoing had not been transcribed] the life that I lead doesn't, doesn't permit it, I don't have this uhhhhh [pause] how can can I tell you (how can I get it across to you) [cut off by interviewer]?

After the respondent's emphasis on the virtures and pleasures of a large kin network, the interviewer's direct question about "the best size for a family" led the respondent to state that the present number of children would be satisfactory. When asked why she did not have only two rather than the actual seven, plus those who have died, the respondent expressed herself only with difficulty. The ensuing dialogue ("Because doesn't, because it doesn't [laughing also], how can I tell you (how can I make it clear to you) the life that I lead doesn't, doesn't permit it . . .") is important insofar as it reveals the difficulties of capturing "the actor's point of view."

12. INTERVIEWER. What are you trying to say (what do you mean) one doesn't, one doesn't have to uhhh?

RESPONDENT. I don't have the peacefulness (peace and quiet), I don't have the harmony (satisfaction), the (this) uhhh, the (this) peace and quiet (tranquillity), the years that one carries (the burden of one's age) . . . [cut off by interviewer].

INTERVIEWER. Right, right [pause], so that is why you have more kids than you really ought to have? [the foregoing was not transcribed by the interviewer.]

RESPONDENT. [in a low voice] And (the) other (reasons) is that I was also unlucky (luck was not with me), so that [voice trails off and the interviewer jumps in with:]

INTERVIEWER. Now for your husband, what do you think is the ideal size? What is the ideal family size? How many kids (slight pause) do you think he wants (prefers)? [The actual question should be: "What is the (an) ideal family size for your husband?"] (FA 195 MU 115-37)

RESPONDENT. If it were left up to him? /INTERVIEWER: Yes./ a dozen.

INTERVIEWER. A dozen? How do you know this is the way he thinks?

RESPONDENT. Because he has told me so (this).

INTERVIEWER. Ah, is that right?

RESPONDENTS Uh (it is) his joy (is) if I had had 12 children, the 12, the 12 if I had them (if I could produce them). [not clear here] . . . this . . . craziness that he had with them (this fondness that he had for them) . (They could have whatever they want) or (He could have whatever problem), whatever dispute (argument, disagreement) with me, but the children . . . [the interviewer then jumps in, changing the direction of the questioning.]

The respondent returned to complaints registered earlier in the interview about family size, but used more general terms to express herself: "I don't have the peacefulness (peace and quiet) , I don't have the harmony (satisfaction)" and earlier, "the life that I lead doesn't, doesn't permit it. . . ." But the interviewer's apparent contradiction—"Right, right, (pause) so that is why you have more kids than you really ought to have?"—comes just when the respondent's remarks perhaps suggest that she, and especially her husband, had desired even more children but because life had not been pleasant and still was difficult, this wish had not been fulfilled. The interviewer's prompting phrase (". . . that is why you have more kids than you really ought to have") did not appear to be linked to her question about why the respondent had had more than two, because the respondent seemed to have altered the latter question; that is, she apparently *responded* to the question: "Why did you not have *more* children than you now have?", although of course this was not asked. The reply was a searching attempt to describe life's difficulties. The interviewer perhaps recognized a shift in interpretation and seemed to be trying to turn the complaint about how difficult life is ("I don't have the peacefulness (peace and quiet)") into a response fitting her original question—namely, why had the woman not restricted herself to two children? The response, nevertheless can be taken to be an indication of why no more than the present number of children were produced. This seems very confusing. Was the interviewer saying that the woman had had more children than she wanted because life had been so miserable (and having more children softens this burden?) , while the woman was saying that she would have had *more* children if life had not been so miserable for her? The interviewer did not pursue the matter further but shifted to the husband's views.

I find the confusion instructive. My fascination stems from the dialogue itself and its apparent disjunctiveness—the absence of a smooth question and answer format . . . the way the participants seemed to be talking past each other. Interviewing and many everyday conversations (particularly family) always seems to contain disjunctiveness, coupled with the tendency of participants to talk past one another. To reduce this information by a simple coding operation destroys the constructive (normative) qualities of everyday accounts about experiences.

The respondent's remarks about the husband's interest in having 12 children implied a devotion to the youngsters that apparently did not carry over to the wife's miserable life. The interviewer asked how the respondent "knew" that the husband would have preferred a dozen children, but the response was not probed or challenged; thus we do not learn about the occasions on which such discussions took place and how the conversations unfolded. The respondent offered details about her husband's devotion to the children, but the interviewer's shift could imply that further elaboration would not be fruitful. Pushing the respondent might reveal that such conversations were rare or consisted of a few flippant remarks in passing.

The Construction of Coding Practices.   Two brief examples of the transformation of ambiguous interview materials into "objective data" serve to close the chapter and to illustrate further the situated or interactional foundation of survey information. The questionnaires utilized were 28 cases obtained from the Buenos Aires Children's Hospital. Most of these cases were chosen arbitrarily from one ward (ward 17). Dr. Florencio Escardó was very generous in allowing us to approach the mothers of children on this ward in the hope of locating families from very low income areas of the city—the *villas miserias* or shantytowns. The mothers were sleeping on the ward to be with their babies. Most of them were from the north of Argentina and would be described by many Argentines as *"cabecitas negras"* or "black heads." As indicated in a previous chapter, the term *"cabecitas negras"* is derogatory and carries many of the implications of racial prejudice found in the United States. The regular sampling procedures did not produce many families representing this group, but the Children's Hospital sample provided a source of information on women with common-law marriages, living under conditions of very poor sanitation and nutrition. The overall educational level was quite low, and some of the women had no schooling at all. The men invariably were manual laborers and the women servants in private homes. If the reported information on number of children can be believed, however, the fertility level did not differ appreciably from the rest of the sample.

I decided to use the Children's Hospital cases to illustrate the problems of coding rather than including them in the regular sample. Because these cases were outside the regular sample, I assumed that some readers would object to finding them in a traditional analysis. Cases of extreme poverty are difficult to obtain by the usual sampling procedures because of the locations involved and because gaining access to the families in shantytowns is never easy—most of the people complain about prying visits from public health officials, researchers, municipal officials, and the police who come to ask "stupid" questions.

To begin the discussion of coding problems, I want to illustrate how problematic a category like "marital status" can be under different circumstances. For example, a man who has a wife and children may be carrying on an extramarital affair from which additional offsprings have resulted. An interviewer with a fixed-choice questionnaire that is to be completed in 50 minutes is not likely to obtain adequate information about extramarital relationships.

But things can be more complicated. As an example, let us consider a male companion of one of the women interviewed. At first we assumed that he was the woman's husband. The couple's language seemed to be matter of fact—the woman spoke of "my husband" and the man spoke of "my wife." The husband was described as timid and the wife as pushing him into the interview, and at times urging him to answer particular questions. The interviewer's impression was that the male respondent was very nervous and found it quite difficult to express himself. Many responses were highly condensed and probes were seldom useful. The man was asked how many women he had lived with, and his replies seemed to be fairly clear at first. He talked specifically about three women, the last being his present wife; but his initial response was that he had gone out with many women. Although the description of each woman seemed to imply a serial order to his affairs, the interviewer noticed considerable overlap in the clock-time periods mentioned indirectly. It appeared that he had been picking fruit in the province of Entre Rios and then in the delta of Buenos Aires province and therefore was often away from "home." But "home" was never clarified in this context. The interviewer decided that he had met the other two women while away from his present wife (or while he was going out steadily with her). The interviewer also concluded that the respondent had lived with each of the two women in a *ranchito* or shack (of the sort found in shantytowns) that resembles the huts typical of rural areas. As I began reading the interview schedule, I found the question–answer sequence confusing. Only when I came to the interviewer's appraisal of the respondent's affairs could I read her account as "reasonable." My attempts to understand the interview material led me to code the man as having had three marriages, but the schedule does not reveal the legal status of any of these unions. The husband implied that he might have made one of the women (not his present wife) pregnant, although he broke up with her before he could be certain and did not see her again. I tried to decide how many women the respondent had lived with, and whether I could accept the interviewer's estimate that he had pursued these affairs while living with or going with his present wife. Written details indicated that all probing questions caused the respondent to gesticulate—grabbing his face, for example, or closing his eyes as if coping with the thoughts the questions evoked. At times the respondent seemed to be so troubled by a question (e.g., "Do you ever talk to your wife about sexual relations?") that he would not say anything for a while, and then "Put down 'yes' and nothing more."

The interviewer's comments about the deportment of the respondent, and the apparently managed and tortuous types of expression he provided, continually stimulated my thoughts about coding the different items. But I had to put my thoughts into written form that would reflect the code established, for a random type of expression would make it difficult to settle on the condensed coding outcomes necessary for cross-tabulation. My wife and I divided the chore of coding the responses, and we found that our running commentaries of the thoughts that occurred to use while attempting to code each item made it hard to settle on a clear-cut choice of one among four or five outcomes. The coding operation involved the disposition of ambiguous, vague, and often contradictory responses into a format permitting cross-tabulation. A coder presumably would avoid this difficulty if he had to deal only with fixed-choice questions. But each coding operation's open-ended questions forced us to make "reasonable" decisions within "reasonable" real-time limits—which could mean anywhere from a few seconds to perhaps a quarter-hour, depending on one's mood, how previous questions had been coded, how tired one felt, and so on. Our personal experience of the time we felt had elapsed while coding influenced how we would discuss the real-time involved. Thus if we felt tired or it was close to lunch or late in the afternoon or night, our experience with an item could seem endless while the actual real-time may have been a matter of minutes or seconds.

The problem of determining when to cut off a respondent and go on to the next question, which has been cited throughout the book, remains one of the interviewer–researcher's most difficult tasks in connection with making claims about the adequacy of his materials or data. But the reasonableness of a participant's remarks or those of a partner in conversation are fused with one's experienced and real-time conceptions of appropriateness vis-à-vis the frequency of utterances, their content, the sense of an unfolding context, future considerations, and the like. Such experienced and real-time conceptions constitute the structure of social interaction. However, the structure of temporal experiences during social interaction is often fortuitous and not readily amenable to description or mapping out in all social exchanges, whether we call them interviews, experiments, conversations, or coding operations.

Our coding practices, therefore, recreate circumstances similar to those that produced the information being coded, because the coder begins to locate the responses in a frame of reference broader than that suggested by the coding rules supplied him. If he knows something about what preceded an item, he may link the former information to the item being coded despite little or no evidence that a relationship exists. But the most important elements are the coder's understanding of the local culture and his thoughts about various activities; the latter, in particular, recreate the kinds of language and non-verbal activities that might have produced the action scenes presumably indexed by the responses. But the routine character of these thoughts and the language employed to represent them are not "obvious" events. The normative or typified structure of verbal and nonverbal materials, which contains a tacit guarantee that the project will not fail, also discloses findings that justify the project's existence. The coder is forced into thinking about events that could make visible the activities indexed by the responses. This means creating or constructing action scenes that would "make sense" out of the condensed information available, thus providing the coder with ethnographic particulars that have been diluted by the interview schedule. The language and thought available to the coder presuppose a native's view of interaction routines and become a critical resource for assuring the positive outcome of the study.

Let me illustrate what I have said with a concrete example concerning the male respondent just mentioned. In reading a response to a question about this individual's knowledge of contraceptives, I neglected to consider that the question itself provided the respondent with a framework in which such devices or methods appeared as known objects or events in an obvious world, which interviewer and respondent are presumed to know in common. The original question asked what a woman should do if she does not want to have children or feels she has all she wants. The respondent answered "take care of herself (be careful) ." When the interviewer reformulated the question, asking whether the respondent knew about contraceptives and their use, the man said that he did not know about contraceptives for males. Had he heard about a woman placing something inside herself before having sexual relations with her husband? According to the interviewer's notes, he replied that he knew about the diaphragm because he had heard someone talk about it. Did he know where contraceptives could be obtained? This series of questions was not recorded verbatim, however, thus we do not know precisely what was asked or what was given (or taken to be given) in response. The interviewer has reconstructed the accounts for us. The interviewer may have supplied the term "diaphragm."

My thinking went as follows: the respondent did not appear to know anything about contraceptives; yet if I am to believe the interviewer's account, he seemed to know something. Otherwise, he could not have (a) denied knowledge of male contraceptives and yet (b) seem to be aware of the existence and function of "diaphragms" in response to a perhaps prompted question about something that women place inside themselves. We have no information about the circumstances under which he could have ". . . heard someone talk about" the diaphragm. We could infer that he did not know about male contraceptives, yet was aware of something the interviewer called a "diaphragm." But inasmuch as the dialogue is not recorded verbatim, we cannot reconstruct with certainty the questions as they were posed. The questions may have been posed one after the other because of the husband's typical unresponsiveness, noted earlier. The hint about ". . . something you place inside" may have been linked to something overheard but not understood at the time by the respondent. Thus the respondent may have acquired new information about contraceptives, or he may have clarified old information because of the interview. But how do I code the responses? In coding categories, we can merely record whether the respondent has "heard about" one or more methods, and proceed to allow for specific methods. Presumed knowledge about contraceptives, especially if this knowledge is in whole or in part created by the interview itself, does not provide the information we actually seek if our interests are only substantive. We would want to know how the respondent became familiar with the methods, the conditions of his obtaining and using the contraceptives, and his conceptions about the significance of their use.

Conclusion. For some couples obtaining and using contraceptives may be so routine a matter that it is not discussed. The central difficulty for the interviewer may be in eliciting comparative information regarding how often and under what circumstances sexual activity takes place. In other families, the acquisition and use of contraceptives may be rather unlikely or highly problematic. But in either case our procedures for claiming knowledge about the acquaintance, acquisition, and use of contraceptives for different segments of the population may never capture the changing day-to-day circumstances surrounding sexual practices and the conditions governing the actual use of contraceptives. The traditional study of fertility is constrained by theories and methods for eliciting information that are divorced from routine family living.

APPENDIX. Spanish Version of Interview Materials

1. Q: ¿Qué cree Ud. que una joven debería saber acerca de relaciones sexuales (¿me entiende?) antes de empezar a salir con un hombre? (FA 115 MU 195-28) (¿Qué tipo de cosas debería conocer una chica, no es cierto, cuando empieza a [pause] antes de salir con un muchacho, sobre ese problema, sobre el problema de relaciones sexuales?) [The interviewer repeated the question but changed it slightly.]

   A: Eh, ¿qué puede ser yo?

   Q: Claro, ¿por tu misma experiencia, no? es decir [not in original transcription.] [Notice shift to familiar form.]

   A: Yo saldría con esa, ¿esa desconfianza [pause] no?

   Q: Aha. Pensand . . . [she changes her remarks before completing the word.] si por, ¿por qué desconfianza, no?

   A: Por qué en realidad uno no conoce la persona, porque uno lo conoce así no más. Uno tiene que conocerse a fondo hasta que se llegue ese momento /INTERVIEWER: Claro/ o que intención hay.

2. Q: Ahora, del problema concreto, del problema de relaciones sexuales, ¿qué debería conocer una chica antes de empezar a salir con muchachos?

   A: Y [pause] el problema que tendría que tener es de, de saber que intenciones tiene esa persona.

   Q: [repeating the last five words] ¿Qué intenciones tiene esa persona? Ahora las chicas con quienes Ud. se crió, ¿cómo se enteraron, acerca del problema de las relaciones sexuales entre el hombre y la mujer? (FA 115 MU 195-28a) (¿Ud. se acuerda? ¿Cómo se enteró Ud. misma?)

A: Yo le voy a decir que yo tuve poco, pocas amistades, pocas amigas, tuve yo. /INTERVIEWER: aha./ Yo sí lo hice, lo hice sola hasta actualmente. A mí me viene cualquiera persona que a mi pide una expicación si se la puede dar, se la doy, si no, no se la doy porque no sé lo que puede /INTERVIEWERS *Claro.*/ ¿contener eso, no? Pero soy una persona que soy poco amiga de tener amigas. Ni ir de visita de ninguna clase a ningún lado.

Q: ¿Entonces cómo Ud. se llegó a enterar de este problema? [The original question was: ¿Como se enteró Ud.?] (FA 115 MU 195-28b) (¿Como se llegó de enterar Ud. del problema?) [Cut off by the respondent.]

A: Por medio de que yo sentía la, las patronas que hablaban, o me aconsejaban, este te conviene, el otro no te conviene. [pause] Así estando yo teniendo hijos, me decía este hombre no te conviene por *h* o *b*, los pocos pesos que vos tenés te los lleva.

3. Q: ¿Ahora con qué frecuencia cree Ud. que una persona necesita tener relaciones? [The question should have been: "¿Con qué frecuencia cree Ud. que una persona necesita tener relaciones sexuales para ser feliz?" (FA 115 MU 195-28i)] [The prior discussion was about sexual relations and I am assuming that this was obvious to both respondent and interviewer. The answer certainly implies this interpretation.]

A: Y por la misma naturaleza.

Q: Ahora, claro, ahora con qué frecuencia, si tomamos como base una semana, por ejemplo, o un mes, cuántas veces cree Ud. qué al mes por ejemplo, necesita tener relaciones, una persona par vivir normalmente, en fin. ¿Toma como base una semana, qué le parece mejor, qué un mes? ¿Y cuántas veces en la semana? [mumble here trailing off.]

A: ¿Hacer uso dice Ud.? [This is the interviewer's transcription. I cannot hear this clearly from the tape.]

Q: Sí, sí, sí. [not in transcript.]

A: Y depende, puede ser todos los días, o puede ser cada tres días, cada cuatro días.

Q: Claro. Depende de la persona, dice Ud.

A: Logic [the respondent cuts herself off before completing "Logico."] Puede ser, y Ud. no puede decir también.

Q: Claro, claro, ¿Yo hablaba así con señoras que me [decían a veces—pause] me daban una alta frecuencia, no? me daban [cut off by respondent]. . . .

4. A: Ahí tiene mi marido así como lo ve, la edad que tiene, si por el fuera todas las noches. A mí me cansa.

Q: Claro, claro. [not in transcript.]

A: Ya el otro no (el otro) fal . . . faltaba seis meses, tres meses y [pause]—[trailing low voice not audible for about three words.] [Both began to speak simultaneously] . . . si fuera todas las noches, señora, todas las noches (y no puede ser)

Q: Así como venía cansao (cansado) [and the voice trails off].

A: [Cutting off the interviewer:] El no le interesa, así, todavía si yo le atiendo me dice que no tengo algo por ahí y no puede ser. Si la edad misma que uno tiene no le permite. Cada tres dias, cada cuatro, cada seis, o cada semana es lo más.

5. Q: Eso es un. . . . [I cannot decipher the last two words.]

A: Sí, Yo lo digo por [pause] la edad que uno tiene, en fin [both talking at once and a few words are lost] ahora Ud. ya es una chica mas joven /INTERVIEWER: claro,/, ¿una señora que en fin que ya, no?

Q: Sí, sí, sí. Bueno, ¿y así todo, también, la [pause] no puede ser así todas las noches, no? No puede ser. [The respondent breaks in almost simultaneously as the interviewer produces these last three words, and for a few moments they both talk at the same time.]

A: No, no, no puede ser, pero [pause] el médico le ha dicho al él, el mismo médico [then two inaudible words] le ha dicho que es muy fuerte de /Interviewer breaks in with "claro, claro."/ naturaleza. /INTERVIEWER: claro, claro./ Come bien! Chupa bien!

Q: Entonces está bien dispuesto siempre.

6. Q: [The next question should have been: "¿Habla Ud. alguna vez con su marido acerca de relaciones sexuales?" The interviewer proceeded as follows:] Ahora, este [the next three words are not clear and the interviewer seems to be having trouble deciding how to formulate the question], yo le voy a preguntar ahora ¿si Ud. habla así alguna vez con su marido acerca de [pause], se acuerda de aquelos problemas que hablábamos ayer? De [pause] de la frecuencia, de cuantas veces Ud. hacía uso [pause], de esos problemas que nosotros hablábamos ayer. ¿Ud. los habla con él? (FA 195 MU 115-31)

A: Sí.

Q: ¿Qué, de qué tipo de cosas, por ejemplo, Ud. le habla a él? (FA 195 MU 115-31a)

A: Me dice ¿de este matrimonio? [This is not clear and the interviewer did not transcribe "este matrimonio" but left it blank. The tape is very difficult to understand.]

Q: Ah, sí y que le dice Ud. a él de esto, o él a Ud. de eso?

A: En lo que me dice que [pause] que ese es el camino de una persona.

7. Q: ¿Matrimonios que no tengan chicos, Ud. conoce señora? [There is a pause here and just as the respondent begins to say something she is cut off by the interviewer with:] Aparte de ese que me contaba recién, se acuerda de la chica ella, aparte /Respondent tries to say something here but is cut off by interviewer/ ... aparte de esa conoce otro matrimonio que no tienen chicos /Resp.: sí, cómo no/ ¿por qué no tienen, que le parece a Ud.? [The question should have been: "¿Conoce Ud. matrimonios que no tengan hijos?"] (FA 195 MU 115-33)

A: Y no tienen porque esta, la señora está enferma o está enfermo el hombre.

8. Q: Ah, por eso no tienen." [Not transcribed by interviewer.] Ahora, ¿matrimonios así que tengan uno o dos chicos, conoce Ud.? /RESPONDENT: Sí, conozco./ Ahora ¿por qué no tienen más que uno, por ejemplo? (FA 195 MU 115-34)

A: Y, por la vida como está de cara, no se quieren cargar también de criaturas. ¿Por qué si compran un kilo de pan, a cuánto está el kilo de pan, señora? ¿Compran un litro de leche, si son dos por qué se va a cargar de uno hoy [The interviewer transcribed this as *cargar* uno hoy.], otro mañana, otro pasado, y qué hace esa gente?

Q: Claro, claro, claro, claro. [voice trailing off]

A: Se pasan de debilidad esos inocentes.

Q: Así, ¿que tienen uno y paran?

A: Y [drawn out] lógico, yo haría otro tanto. Yo con dos, ni que me vinieran [something garbled] los quisiera.

9. Q: Claro. Ahora en general, ¿qué le parece a Ud. [the *Usted* was not completed], quiénes les gusta más una familia grande, a los hombres o a las mujeres? ¿Una familia con muchos chicos, a quiénes le gusta más?

A: Y si se llevan bien en el matrimonio yo creo que tanto el hombre cómo la mujer, es, es una cosa que [pause] ¿es lindo no? /INTER-

VIEWER: claro/ en realidad es lindo, porque es lindo ver [pause] una mesa que haga, póngale 10, 12 chicos, cómo fuímos nosotros 17.

A: Es lindo. En la casa de [this word is drawn out as part of a pause] también de mi marido [next word not clear if it is "allí" or "de"] en Tucumán, también ¿cuántos chicos eran?

Q: ¿Era una mesa que, Dios mío, no?

10. Q: Tus padres [the tape becomes unintelligible for a few words here, and the interviewer did not bother to transcribe them] de ver esas cosas. [At this point the respondent cut in and the two spoke simultaneously until the interviewer gave way.]

A: . . . después vienen grandes y después están los padres, los abuelos, los bisabuelos, los nietos, los vinietos, es, es una sola [cut off by interviewer].

Q: Es una familia muy, muy numerosa. /RESPONDENT: eh?/ familia . . . [Both begin speaking simultaneously and it is difficult to disentangle their remarks.]

A: . . . pero para [pause] una madre, a mí me parece, un padre eso es algo grande en la vida /INTERVIEWER: claro/ de ver con har monía [the next utterance was said simultaneously with the interviewer cutting in with "ahora par Ud."] ¿qué se yo?

11. Q: Ahora para Ud. así, ¿cuál cree que es el mejor tamaño, de una familia? [actual question: "¿Cuál cree Ud. que es el mejor tamaño de una familia?' ' (FA 195 MU 115-36)] Es decir, ¿que cantidad de hijos [pause] tendría que tener para Ud.?

A: Yo me, yo le digo sinceramente [not too clear, but the respondent seems to be laughing slightly as if to convey the impression she is hesitant because of revealing a kind of minor confession], yo me conformo con esto que tengo y nada más.

Q: ¿Nada más que eso no? [Not transcribed by interviewer.]

A: Nada, nada.

Q: Ahora [the interviewer seems to be laughing—I cannot tell whether in response to the solemn way in which the respondent said "nada, nada" or whether perhaps she was embarrassed by the next question], ¿por qué Ud. no tuvo dos en vez de tener, cuanto tuvo Ud.? ehhh, son cinco [they both said "cinco" simultaneously] no siete [they both said "siete" at the same time].

A: Siete, siete, bueno, pero los demás muertos.

Q: Claro, claro, claro [pause] ¿por qué no tuvo Ud. entonces [laughing slightly again] nada más que dos?

A: Por qué no, por qué no la [laughing also], cómo le puedo decir [all the foregoing had not been transcribed] la vida que llevo, no, no me le permite, no tengo esaaa [pause] cómo le puede decir . . . [cut off by the interviewer here].

12. Q:¿ Que quiere decir Ud., no no tiene que, ehhh?

A: No tengo tranquilidad, no tengo harmonía, ese, ehh, esa tranquilidad, los años que uno lleva . . . [cut off by interviewer].

Q: Claro, claro [pause], ¿así es por eso que Ud. tiene más chicos de los que en realidad tendría que tener? [The foregoing was not transcribed by the interviewer.]

A: [in a low voice] Y otra que tampoco tuve suerte, así que . . . [voice trails off and the interviewer jumps in with:]

Q: Ahora para su marido, ¿cuál cree que es tamaño ideal Ud.? ¿con [or "que es"] el tamaño ideal de familia? ¿Qué cantidad de chicos [slight pause] cree que él quiere?" [The actual question should be: "¿Cuál es el tamaño ideal de una familia para su marido?" (FA 195 MU 115-37)]

A: ¿Si por él fuera? /Inter.: Sí/ una docena.

Q: Una docena? ¿Cómo sabe Ud. que él piensa así?

A: Porque me lo ha dicho.

Q: Ah, ¿sí?

A: Eh la alegría de él si yo hubiera tenido 12 hijos, los 12, los 12 se los cría [not clear here] . . . eso . . . locura que tenía con ellos. ¿Cualquier cosa puede tener, cualquirer disputa conmigo, pero los hijos? [The interviewer then jumps in.]

CHAPTER 10

AN ALTERNATE APPROACH TO FIELD RESEARCH

Sociologists cannot escape talking to respondents or giving them verbal materials that cognitively recreate face-to-face experiences with others. Despite the continual attempts by researchers to extract simple quantitative findings from qualitative questioning, we cannot avoid the complex social processes that produce sociological information. Attempts to use statistical procedures to mask the qualitative judgments inherent in everyday social structures can create a misleading sense of quantitative inference. Quantification is not achieved by a brute force transformation of everyday language into numeric forms that will permit the use of correlation techniques. If we are to aspire to realistic inferences about social structure, we must possess a model of the actor's movements, his thinking, and his perception and use of language in socially defined settings. Such a model does not emerge from research procedures and analysis that either dismiss or take for granted the structure of everyday communication.

In the present work I have not implemented an alternate strategy for the gathering and analysis of social interaction information; rather, I have indicated how survey materials can be subjected to other interpretations that challenge inferences made from traditional research procedures. In this final chapter, I briefly introduce an alternate strategy that has been emerging (in the wake of the present fertility study) in recent research with doctoral students.

The alternate strategy is merely a first step in achieving control over the elicitation and analysis of information on social processes. The strategy has roots in philosophical studies of ordinary language, as well as in structural and transformational linguistics, cognitive psychology,

developmental psycholinguistics, and linguistically oriented anthropological works on componential analysis and the ethnography of speaking. One issue I want to address deals with the organization of verbal
and nonverbal displays in everyday life as these activities can be said to
depict belief systems and routine or ceremonial activities. Another topic
is comprised of the various ways in which the actor's or respondent's
thinking and experiences are elicited and represented by the investigator.
Research (Cicourel 1973) on these issues has shown that different interpretations of the "same" event or object by the same or different respondents occur routinely, and this circumstances raises serious questions
about the credibility of materials obtained from instruments that employ
only one narrow interrogative procedure or a traditional form of participant observation from "within" a group by one researcher.

Sociologists always use standardized sentences when constructing questionnaire items. These sentences are usually followed by fixed-choice
alternatives that facilitate their completion and their coding and analysis.
Each sentence is presumed to be self-contained and pretested with respect
to its theoretical and substantive meaning. The context of communication
is assumed to be controlled through standardized questions and neutral
presentation of each item, although researchers have long acknowledged
that interviewer bias is always present in some form. Recent work on
sociolinguistics forces us to recognize that a much broader context is
needed for understanding single or model sentences. Any particular
sentence implies other information tacitly tied to the questionnaire item.
The significance of a question may not be recognized by the respondent
until several items later, but he may fail to advise the interviewer that
he now better understands a previous item, but may not wish to verbalize
this information. Hence each sentence must be located against a background of ethnographic and behavioral particulars that often remains
an unspoken feature of the interview, yet is an integral part of any
response. Since ethnographic and behavioral particulars interact with
the unfolding context of the interview itself, the respective meanings of
a question and of a response are sharply constrained by a fixed-choice
set of alternatives.

Research on language structure and use (Cicourel 1973), on language
use in classroom and testing situations (Cicourel et al. in press), and
with encounter groups (Shumsky 1972) has revealed how subjects alter
their interpretations of events they had experienced and described previously to a researcher. The issue of what constitutes the data base becomes problematic and is contingent on the setting, the informational

(or stimulus) particulars the respondent generates and is permitted to witness, and the respondent's memory and reorganization of prior experiences. The selective attention possible at the time of interrogation interacts with the memory stimulated by an actual setting. The problem can be posed as follows: what do we do about these exigencies?

We must first recognize that utterances elicited on a particular occasion cannot be given self-evident status. This point may seem obvious for attitudinal information, but it can be valid for seemingly concrete informational details (e.g., occupation), as well. Within an organization, the particular occupant of a position may be accorded minimal respect by his peers. The abstract meaning assigned to the occupation by a sample survey of occupational prestige, however, becomes equivocal if the respondents' knowledge of occupations is not a variable features of the study. Similarly, a person's income is always compromised by obligations and tastes that hinder the making of "objective" inferences about life style. Correlational studies of educational success and race and ethnicity do not capture the consequences of the day-to-day emotional strain and cognitive activities that take place in the classroom and during testing sessions.

One way of facing the problem of the occasionality of verbal expressions is in creating circumstances whereby the same and different respondents react to information obtained on a previous occasion. The role of attention and memory becomes paramount, as does the respondent's ability to utilize specific lexical items or vocabularies. I have termed this procedure "indefinite triangulation" to emphasize that no fixed number of accounts will produce an ideal "satisfactory" response, yet researchers obviously can settle on materials they will justify within the existing practical circumstances of the research. But there is an important lesson to be learned from the apparent possibility of indefinite accounts. The discrepancies in accounts and their neglect of important nonverbal materials become the focus of attention because the selective attention and memory of human information processing lead to an understanding of persistence and change in normative accounts. The researcher's problem is to make visible to a reader the often unstated decisions resulting in the creation and acceptance of materials labeled "data" and "findings."

Notice that the accounts may satisfy a normative structure that includes a standardized subject-verb-object construction, dictionary entries that correspond to lexical items used, and other similar details; but there will be variations in the substantive interpretation (he sounds "hostile," "it's me again but I'm not sure what I was trying to say," "I sound angrier than I thought I was or meant to be"). Normative accounts are very important for the construction and reification of social structure as "real," but their meaning derives from situated events and their use in any macroanalysis cannot be divorced from the situated experiences of the participants.

Traditional substantive research in sociology and demography fails to specify the interface between an actor's acquisition and use of the social competence necessary to produce the kinds of activities about which he or she is being questioned, and the implementation of the competence presupposed in asking questions and receiving answers. I do not suggest that macrostructure is irrelevant, but that its significance requires a conception of and a commitment to a theory of social or interactional competence. This competence must include consideration of the means by which man's social activities are produced by complex information-processing structures.

The description of macrosocial structures trades on an implicit notion of interactional competence or information processing in socially defined settings. Interactional competence makes conversational exchanges and everyday decisions possible, and these exchanges and decisions are the basis for the researcher's claims to substantive knowledge. Unless we know something about the interface between interactional competence and social exhanges, we cannot assess the significance of substantive knowledge. Social exchanges occur in ethnographic settings; hence we need a strategy that simultaneously represents the context and seeks control over information elicited and used.

Because ethnographic context is fundamental, to every interviewing strategy this context must be indexed in the analysis of responses. The interviewing strategy I taught my interviewers during the present study was based on two broadly related principles. First, the interviewer was instructed to encourage the respondent to relate descriptive examples from recent experiences that would be likely to stimulate the memory of the occasion which the questions were designed to clarify. Second, I advised the use of probes that would continually press for details about past experiences to stimulate a respondent's experiences of the setting and its unfolding character. The use of probes can make a respondent angry or uncomfortable because it forces him to "work at" his responses, in a way that tends to preclude flippant or evasive, abstract answers.

We have found it useful (Cicourel 1973) to go beyond the strategies just outlined by returning at a later date and showing the transcript to to the respondent, who is asked to clarify responses and to comment on his or her understanding of the questions. Another variation involves two tape recorders—one plays the original interview, which the respondent follows by means of the transcript, and the second machine tapes the respondent's reaction to the previous dialogue. If video recordings have been made, we have found it convenient first to present a rerun of the transcript and audio version of the exchange or test situation, then to return to show the videotape. This procedure allows the researcher to produce several analyses of the "same" exchange or test and to keep track of how he elicited and interpreted different versions of the respondent's remarks.

In still another variation, we play the audio tape for respondents, to elicit their views of other exchanges. Having the respondents serve as temporary research assistants is an excellent way of gaining insight into the layman's everyday reasoning that precedes responses; it also indicates how fortuitous many responses are. We have also used the techniques of simulating an interview and exposing the results to respondents, to show how interviewers interpret and represent different respondents. Here we are concerned with assigning to questions and responses a level of credibility that can be justified in the analysis of materials.

In a recent study of language use in classroom and testing settings (cf. Mehan's chapter in Cicourel, et al. in press), we presented to teachers materials derived from transcripts of classroom and testing interaction or interviews. The transcripts were created from the soundtracks of audio- or videotapes recorded in classrooms, homes, and meetings. We used videotapes to make explicit some of the conditions that are masked in traditional sociological and educational psychological research, where surveys, tests, and field and interview notes are the basis for presenting findings. The audiovisual materials can help clarify the basis for many of the routine measurement decisions made in social and behavioral science research.

Our equipment was a tripod-mounted Sony with a wide-angle lens camera that is part of a Sony model AV 3600 half-inch videorecorder. The television monitor used in the recording enabled us to allow children to view themselves after their participation; we could also interview teachers and testers about the lessons and tests they gave us, as outlined previously in describing the "indefinite triangulation" procedure. The camera was set up in full view of the participants; thus its presence was explicit and could become a routine part of the already-familiar setting. However, having the video equipment fully visible to the participants limited the extent to which we could capture certain settings, depending on the lesson of the day or the kind of activities that different groups performed. Locating the recipient of a teacher's or child's remarks often required highly professional camera movements, while individual voices were often unidentified if the camera was focused only on one part of the room.

The use of video equipment did not eliminate the usual problems of field research whereby the selective attention of the researcher's observations and notes condense severely the interactional settings available for study. But the equipment enabled us to focus on many details of interaction that are missed in participant observation studies and simultaneously made us aware of the enormous problems of describing what appeared to be routine classroom and testing activities. Even with several researchers available and necessary for video recording and independent observations and field notes, it became obvious to us that traditional field studies cannot capture the subtleties of (a) emergent social interaction and (b) the assembling of accounts about the emergent setting that are produced by participants during and after an episode.

We became acutely aware of the difficulties of assembling a transcript from the videotapes because of the disjuncture between what can be seen and what is heard. Having the audio part of the videotape copied for transcription with a heavy-duty tape recorder makes it easier to assemble a transcript, but this procedure can distort the meaning of the materials, depending on how one decides to analyze the transcript. Paying close attention to the video activities means that the researcher using a linguistic or conversational data base will ignore many of the important features of the picture that are necessary for understanding the structure of the interactional scene. Having observed the video-recorded scene, the observer will continually add information from his memory of the setting to enhance or alter the impression evoked by the video screen or transcript. But we were all selective in the kinds of materials we included or excluded from our analyses of various settings, and, of course, this general problem turns out to be the central issue in arriving at a way of describing a study for readers who were not participants. It is difficult to show how the selectivity of our research accounts simplifies the phenomena addressed while simultaneously providing the impression of "completeness" because of the global nature of the language used.

The use of audiovisual materials provides the reader with a basis for evaluating the researcher's procedures and claims to knowledge, if the assembly of a data base and its analysis come to comprise a problematic feature of the findings reported. In this study we wanted to supply information about the problems of assembling a data base and its analysis, while emphasizing that the substantive problem facing the teacher and tester involves a similiar set of issues. The classroom lesson and the testing situation are either too diffuse or are highly reified settings for making inferences about children's abilities and performances. Our research report attempted to highlight these methodological issues and to address the substantive problems in a format that preserves the contextual quality of routine classroom and testing activities.

I am not concerned merely with the respondent's ability to lie or mislead the interviewer, but with the normal basis for constructing any account of one's activities under a variety of circumstances. If the questions posed have syntactic and semantic structures that are not congruent with those used by a sample of respondents, we have no way of knowing how the respondents processed and retrieved information that would be relevant to the question. An interviewer's paraphrasing of standardized questions is a way of sensing that an item is not appropriately worded or may be irrelevant to the respondent. Everyday conversation involves considerable paraphrasing and rewording of utterances, along with miscellaneous fillers and nonverbal information that furnishes to each participant clues that things are going well—or are being misunderstood, or are annoying.

Our interrogative procedures must be articulated with the ways in which information from different modalities is perceived and stored. Simple question–answer formats cannot handle or anticipate the complexities of human information unless they treat interviews as similar to experimental occasions aimed at revealing the interface between information-processing activities and the production of substantive materials. The interviewer seldom realizes how much information is being taken for granted in his own implementation of the questionnaire.

Moreover, we usually fail to design questions to fit what we think of, or independently examine, as the respondents' life experiences. Our questions are designed to facilitate the coding of the responses and the subsequent assembly of neat tables. It may be impossible to formulate a standardized question that (a) can retrieve desired information, (b) is assumed to be farily well bounded, and (c) will be applicable to a cross section of a population. It is not simply a matter of differences in dialect, although they are important; also to be considered are the ways in which prior information is experienced, stored, retrieved, and modified by the situated circumstances of the interview. Hence we need constant controls over our means of eliciting information, the possible intentions of a question or an answer, and the relation between the information obtained, the ethnographic context of the original experiences, and the interview. We cannot achieve controls unless the interview and (wherever possible) the original experiences are treated as activities to be studied independently of the researcher's substantive interests. We must create circumstances for generating contrasting versions of the "same" information.

There are roughly four ways in which information should be obtained in field studies. Initially there should be participant observation—for example, spending considerable time with a few families, with a particular organization or classroom, or in a single neighborhood. This would be followed by interviewing by way of a standardized format but allowing for restructuring the questions and the use of extensive probes. Tapes of the interviews would be an aid in the independent study of the social processes used in obtaining contrasting substantive perspectives. Although I have not suggested that a traditional survey be included, I realize that many researchers feel that fixed-choice questions are necessary when sampling a large cross section of a population, if valid and representative results are to be obtained. The use of this kind of research instrument can have occasional short-term benefits, but the strategy is motivated more by methodological expediency than by its theoretical sophistication.

The Representational Problem. How we represent what we call information is central to the use of all procedures for the elicitation and analysis of data. Research on memory and attention reveals how difficult it is to recall details accurately over real time. When we experiment with the phenomenon of the transmission of rumors, it is evident that important alterations occur in "information." This problem in information processing and representation is not addressed seriously by researchers who advocate participant observation, and it is ignored by survey researchers when eliciting information from respondents. Every account is a historical document because selective attention and memory are involved and because several sensory modalities are being utilized but only partially represented by the verbal expressions we call data. Traditional conceptions of social structure at the level of macroanalysis are rather abstract, beginning with naïve verbal observations or accounts and reports of "objective social facts." Endowing such information with the status of "objective data" eliminates many complex problems and provides a simplified view of topics such as "the American occupational structure," "differential fertility," or "attitudes toward abortion."

Eliciting and organizing information is a creative activity that articulates situated meaning structures with information stored in memory. Our verbal constructions (be they opinions, attitudes, or descriptions of such circumstances as occupations, level of education, number of children, or amount of income earned) do not adequately index various forms of information recognized, received, processed, and intended in the descriptive forms we actually express.

With the alternate conception of field research I have outlined in this brief chapter, all elicitation procedures and coding must be subjected to controlled reinterpretation by the same and different respondents and coders. Reinterpretation by the same and different respondents and coders is not designed merely to check on the reliability of the responses and coding, but to reveal how such constructions are accomplished and to make visible elements of interactional competence and cognitive processes that are an integral part of what is to be called "objective social facts" or data. Forcing coders to justify their ad hoc operations discloses how historicized events are created by selective attention to situated particulars.

An ethnographic foundation is essential for locating elicited material on everyday exchanges such as those occurring in offices, classrooms, and families, or in patient–physician relationships. Ethnographic information commits the researcher to reveal details about the interaction that produces outcomes he treats as data. The interactional processes of elicitation embellish the ethnographic descriptive particulars to expose the respondent's use of language and nonverbal communication. The respondent's use of language and nonverbal communication, in turn, can provide clues about his descriptions of past experiences and the activities of others. The elicitation of information permits the researcher access to the respondent's procedures for creating accounts under such conditions that, presumably, the respondent's reflexive self-monitoring of outputs would increase the chances of his idealizing and glossing his experiences. Elicited information must be contrasted with materials secured from the daily workings of individual respondents in the settings in which the activities the researcher seeks to clarify are routinely enacted. It is not easy to obtain permission to leave a tape recorder, much less to utilize a video recording strategy with every conceivable research setting. However, we have found it increasingly easier to gain such permission when the subjects to be studied are given the opportunity to observe or listen to their activities and to offer their criticisms of our interpretations. Hence the controlled indefinite triangulation—whereby respondents can react to their previous accounts or the accounts of others, as well as the interpretations of the researcher—provides conditions for approximating a few experimental controls. Moving from the field setting into the controlled elicitation of information by way of structured interviews, or exposing the respondent to his own accounts or those of others, gives us insight into our constructions and inferences and those of the subjects we study. If we can then return to a field setting and observe and record daily activities, we can better pinpoint the ways in which normative constructions are generated in contingent circumstances.

When only a survey is employed, the foregoing alternate strategy is simulated only indirectly by a few activities—pretests, limited interviews with interviewers and postinterview follow-ups, coder flagging of discrepancies or unusual information, and the like—but these efforts are never studied (and seldom reported) in their own right as central ingredients of the study and of the "findings" presented in tabular and correlational form. Basically, I have tried to determine how members, at different developmental stages in acquiring adult competence and at different stages in the life cycle, make claims to knowledge and treat such claims as grounds for further inference and action. In this book I have examined this and related issues by utilizing traditional methods to study a topic central to sociological interests.

References

Banks, Joseph A., 1954. *Prosperity and Parenthood: A Study of Family Planning Among the Victorian Middle Classes.* London: Routledge & Kegan Paul.

Beshers, James M., 1967. *Population Processes in Social Systems.* New York: Free Press.

Blake, Judith (in collaboration with J. M. Stycos and K. Davis), 1961. *Family Structure in Jamaica.* New York: Free Press.

Blau, Peter, and Otis D. Duncan, 1967. *The American Occupational Structure.* New York: Wiley.

Blau, Peter, and W. R. Scott, 1962. *Formal Organizations.* San Francisco: Chandler.

Canton, Darío, 1965. "Notas sobre las Fuerzas Armadas Argentinos," *Revista Latinoamericana de Sociología,* **3**.

Cicourel, Aaron V., 1964. *Method and Measurement in Sociology.* New York: Free Press.

Cicourel, Aaron V., 1967. "Fertility, Family Planning and the Social Organization of Family Life: Some Methodological Issues," *Journal of Social Issues,* **23** (October), 57–81.

Cicourel, Aaron V., 1968. *The Social Organization of Juvenile Justice.* New York: Wiley.

Cicourel, Aaron V., 1972. "Ethnomethodology," in Thomas A. Sebeok, A. S. Abramson, D. Hymes, H. Rubenstein, E. E. Stankiewicz, and B. Spolsky (eds). *Current Trends in Linguistics,* Vol. 12. The Hague: Mouton.

Cicourel, Aaron V., 1973. *Cognitive Sociology: Language and Meaning in Social Interaction.* New York: Penguin.

Cicourel, A. V., K. Jennings, S. Jennings, K. Leiter, R. Mackay, H. Mehan, and D. Roth, in press. *Language Use in Testing and Classroom Settings.* New York and San Francisco: Academic Press.

Ciria, Alberto, 1964. *Partidos y Poder en la Argentina Moderna 1930–1946.* Buenos Aires: Jorge Alvarez.

Coale, A. J. et al. (eds.), 1965. *Aspects of the Analysis of Family Structure.* Princeton, N.J.: Princeton University Press.

Conde, Roberto Cortés, 1965. "Problemas del Crecimiento Industrial (1870–1914)," in T. Di Tella, G. Germani, J. Graciarena et al. (eds.), *Argentina, Sociedad de Masas.* Buenos Aires: EUDEBA.

Cornblit, Oscar, Ezequiel Gallo, and Alfredo O'Connell, 1965. "La Generación del 80 y su Proyecto: Antecedentes y Consecuencias," in T. Di Tella et al., *Argentina, Sociedad de Masas.*

Davis, Kingsley, 1959. "The Sociology of Demographic Behavior," in R. K. Merton, L. Broom, and L. S. Cottrell, Jr. (eds.), *Sociology Today.* New York: Basic Books.

Davis, Kingsley, 1963. "The Theory of Change and Response in Modern Demographic History," *Population Index*, **29**, no. 4.

Davis, K. and J. Blake, 1956. "Social Structure and Fertility: An Analytic Framework," *Economic Development and Cultural Change*, **4** (April), 211–235.

Di Tella, T. G. Germani, J. Graciarena et al. (ed.) , 1965. *Argentina, Sociedad de Masas*. Buenos Aires: EUDEBA.

Di Tella, Guido and Manuel Zymelman, 1965. "Etapas de Desarrollo Económico Argentino," in T. Di Tella et al., *Argentina, Sociedad de Masas*.

Fallars, L. A., 1965. "A Critique of Marion J. Levy, Jr.'s Argument," in A. J. Coale et al. (eds.), *Aspects of the Analysis of Family Structure*. Princeton, N.J.: Princeton University Press.

Ferrer, Aldo, 1963. *La Economia Argentina*. Mexico-Buenos Aires. Fondo de Cultura Económica.

Frake, Charles, 1961. "The Diagnosis of Disease Among the Subanum of Mindanao," *American Anthropology*, **63**.

Freedman, Ronald, 1963. "Changing Fertility in Taiwan," in R. O. Greep (ed.), *Human Fertility and Population Problems*. Cambridge, Mass.: Schenkman.

Freedman, R., P. K. Whelpton, and A. A. Campbell, 1959. *Family Planning, Sterility, and Population Growth*. New York: McGraw-Hill.

Gallo, Ezequiel and Silvia Sigal, 1965, "La Formación de los Partidos Politicos Contemporaneos: la U.C.R. (1890-1916) ," in T. Di Tella et al., *Argentina, Sociedad Masas*.

Garfinkel, Harold, 1964. "Studies of the Routine Grounds of Everyday Activities," *Social Problems*, **11**, 225–250.

Garfinkel, Harold, 1967. *Studies in Ethnomethodology*. Englewood Cliffs, N.J.: Prentice-Hall.

Germani, Gino, 1962. *Politica y Sociedad en una Época de Transición*. Buenos Aires: Paidos.

Germani, Gino, 1965. "Hacia una Democracia de Masas," in T. Di Tella et al., *Argentina, Sociedad de Masas*.

Goode, William J., 1960. "Norm Commitment and Conformity to Role–Status Obligations," *American Journal of Sociology*, **66**, 246-258.

Goodenough, W., 1957. "Cultural Anthropology and Linguistics," in D. Hymes (ed.), *Language in Culture and Society*. New York: Harper & Row, 1964.

Gumperz, John J. and Jan-Petter Blom, 1971. "Social Meaning in Linguistic Structures: Code Switching in Norway," in Gumperz and Hymes (eds.), *Directions in Sociolinguistics*. New York: Holt, Rinehart, & Winston.

Hawthorne, Geoffrey, 1970. *The Sociology of Fertility*. London: Collier-Macmillan.

Hill, R., J. M. Stycos, and K. Back, 1959. *The Family and Population Control*. Chapel Hill, N.C.: University of North Carolina Press.

Leik, R. K., 1965. " 'Irrelevant' Aspects of Stooge Behavior," *Sociometry*, **28**, 259–271.

Petersen, William, 1961. *Population*. New York: Macmillan.

Rainwater, Lee, 1960. *And the Poor Get Children*. New York: Quadrangle.

Rainwater, Lee, 1965. *Family Design*. Chicago: Aldine.

Romero, José Luis, 1959. *Las Ideas Politicas en Argentina*. Buenos Aires: Fondo de Cultura Económica.

Sacks, Harvey, 1966. *The Search for Help: No One to Turn To*. Unpublished dissertation, Department of Sociology. University of California, Berkeley.

Sacks, Harvey, 1967. Dittoed lectures, University of California, Irvine.

Schneider, David, 1965. "Kinship and Biology," in A. J. Coale et al., *Aspects of the Analysis of Family Structure*.

Schutz, Alfred, 1943. "The Problem of Rationality in the Social World," *Economica*, **10**.

Schutz, Alfred, 1962. *Collected Papers, Vol. I. The Problem of Social Reality*, M. Natanson (ed.). The Hague: Nijhoff.

Schutz, Alfred, 1964. *Collected Papers, Vol. II. Studies in Social Theory*, A. Brodersen (ed.). The Hague: Nijhoff.

Schutz, Alfred, 1966. *Collected Papers*, Vol. III. *Studies in Phenomenological Philosophy*, I. Schultz (ed.). The Hague: Nijhoff.

Shumsky, M., 1972. *Encounter Groups: A Forensic Science*. Ph.D. dissertation, University of California, Santa Barbara.

Scobie, James R., 1964. *Argentina: A City and a Nation*. New York: Oxford University Press.

Stinchcombe, Arthur L., 1968. *Constructing Social Theories*. New York: Harcourt Brace Jovanovich.

Stycos, J. Mayone, 1955. *Family and Fertility in Puerto Rico*. New York: Columbia University Press.

Stycos, J. M. and K. Back, 1964. *The Control of Human Fertility in Jamaica*. Ithaca, N.Y.: Cornell University Press.

Weber, M., 1947. *The Theory of Social and Economic Organization*, trans. by T. Parsons. New York: Free Press.

Westoff, C. F., R. G. Potter, and P. C. Sagi, 1963. *The Third Child*. Princeton, N.J.: Princeton University Press.

Westoff, C. F., R. G. Potter, P. C. Sagi, and E. G. Mishler, 1961. *Family Growth in Metropolitan America*. Princeton, N.J.: Princeton University Press.

Whelpton, P. K. and C. V. Kiser, 1958. "Summary of Chief Findings and Implications for Future Studies," *Milbank Memorial Fund Quarterly*, **36** (July), 282–329.

Wrong, Dennis H., 1967. *Population and Society*, 3rd ed. New York: Random House.

Wyon, John B., 1963. "Field Studies on Fertility of Human Populations," in R. O. Greep (ed.), *Human Fertility and Population Problems*. Cambridge, Mass.: Schenkman.

AUTHOR INDEX

Back, K., 2, 16, 24, 206
Banks, J. A., 24, 205
Beshers, J. M., 16–26, 205
Blake, J., 2, 16, 70–71, 83, 91, 130, 205, 206
Blau, P., 23, 205
Blom, J. P., 54, 206

Campbell, A. A., 25, 206
Canton, Dario, 39, 205
Cicourel, A. V., 14, 20, 196, 198, 199, 205
Ciria, A., 205
Coale, A. J., 205
Conde, R. C., 32, 205
Cornblit, O., 30, 32, 205

Davis, K., 2, 4–8, 205
Di Tella, G., 27
Di Tella, T., 32
Duncan, O. D., 205

Escardó, F., 184

Fallars, L. A., 26, 206
Ferrer, A., 34, 37–38, 206
Frake, C., 21, 206
Framini, A., 56
Freedman, R., 25, 206
Frondizi, A., 36

Gallo, E., 30, 32, 205–206
Gardel, C., 44
Garfinkel, H., 14, 20, 206
Germani, G., 27, 30–31, 36, 38–39, 43, 62, 69, 206
Goode, W. J., 11, 206
Goodenough, W., 21, 206
Graciarena, J., 27, 206
Gumperz, J. J., 54, 206

Hawthorne, G., 206
Hill, R. J., 16, 24, 206

Jennings, K., 196, 205
Jennings, S., 196, 205

Kiser, C. V., 2, 207

Leik, R. K., 85, 206
Leiter, K., 196, 205

MacKay, R., 196, 205
Mehan, H., 196, 199, 205
Mishler, E. G., 3, 207

O'Connell, A., 30, 32, 205

Perón, E. D., 35–40, 81
Perón, J. D., 35–41, 55, 81
Petersen, W., 2, 3, 206
Potter, R. G., 3, 207

Rainwater, L., 2, 16, 206
Romero, J. L., 27, 207
Roth, D. B., 196, 205

Sacks, H., 21, 207
Sagi, P. C., 3
Schneider, D., 74, 207
Schutz, A., 14, 20, 23, 207
Scobie, J. R., 27–28, 32–36, 207
Scott, W. R., 23, 205
Shomsky, M., 196, 207
Sigal, S., 32, 207
Stinchcombe, A. L., 207
Stycos, J. M., 2, 16, 24, 70–71, 91, 130, 207

Torales, P., 43

Vandor, A., 56

Weber, M., 24–25, 207
Westoff, C. F., 3, 207
Whelpton, P. K., 2, 25, 207

Wrong, D. H., 2, 3, 4, 207
Wyon, J. B., 3, 207

Zymelman, M., 32, 206

SUBJECT INDEX

Argentine history, 28–42
  colonial period, 28–29
  economic development, 29–39
  generation of the 80's, 29–32
  immigration, 30–31
  modern period, 33–42
  Peronism, 35–41, 55–59
  political development. 31–41
  Radical party, 33–37
  Yrigoyen, 32–34
Attitudes, 19
  on contraceptives, 131–138
  on family size, 115–118, 128–130
  and fertility, 18–23
  and interview questions, 83–85, 89, 93
    100, 107–108
  about sexual relations, 169–174

Buenos Aires, 42–59
  education, 48–51
  everyday social interaction, 51–54
    language use in daily activities, 51–54
  family life, 54–55, 64–68, 75–83
  labor activities, 55–59
  streets, housing, and services, 44–47, 64–68

Characteristics of the sample studied, 62–71
  family size, 115–118
    and religion, 118–125
    and use of contraceptives, 131–138
  life style, 63–68
  marriage and divorce, 70–72
  rural-urban differences, 69
  socioeconomic status, 63–68
Cognitive sociological view, 12, 20–24
  and rationality, 23
  and typifications by the actor, 23
Comparative research issues, 59–61

Decision-making, 15
  and family planning practices, 15, 26
  and fertility, 15–18
  and modes of orientation, 21–23
  rationality, 15, 18
Demographic theory, 3–11
  and social interaction, 5, 9

Fertility, 1, 2
  and decision-making, 15
  decline in rates, 2, 4–5
  differential, 3
  and everyday family life, 6, 26
  and family size, 115–118, 128–130
  Indianapolis studies of, 2, 24
  and modernization, 25
  in nonindustrialized countries, 3–5
  population problem and, 1
  and religion, 118–125
  and rural conditions, 6–8, 10
  and sexual unions, 91–97, 157–159
  stimulus and response conditions, 4–8
  systems of communication and, 5, 24
  and use of contraceptives, 131–138
  variables affecting rates, 1, 3, 26, 90

Methodological issues, 8–11, 18–21
  alternate field research, 195
    ethnographic context, 198–203
    "indefinite triangulation," 197–204
    memory and attention, 202–203
    use of audio and video tapes, 199–201
  in field studies, 75–83
  influence of the setting on questions asked,
    100–107
  problems of, coding responses, 184–189
    interviewing, 84–89, 93–95, 148–157
    tables without textual materials, 113–139

211

textual analysis of interviews, 141–157
  family size, 142
  use of contraceptives, 145–148

Social interaction, 2, 21–23, 108, 195–203
  and demographic theory, 5, 9–10
  cognitive and linguistic factors, 2
Sociolinguistic features of interviews, 162–184
  alternative interpretations of textual
    material, 165–168, 173–175, 179,
    183–184
  creating an "objective" text, 176–177,
    200–201

cross-modal information, 201
Survey research, 13
  questionnaire defects, 11, 19–21, 89,
    168–169
  social competence of respondent, 198

Table of organization view of society, 11–14
  and demographic transition, 12
  and family organization, 13
  and kinship, 12
  and model of the actor, 13–14
  role, 11–13
  status, 11